SYNERGIZE YOUR HEALTH

THE 6 ELEMENTS TO GREATER VITALITY AND JOY

KRISTY WARE

STOKEPUBLISHING

PRAISE

In *Synergize Your Health* Kristy Ware inspires us to learn how to take better care of ourselves through an engaging mix of client stories, research, and personal examples. Using her elements of self-care, Ware gives us a concrete framework that is 'sticky' and easy to use. For anyone who struggles with taking consistent care of themselves or who is ready to add another layer of self-care to their lives, *Synergize Your Health* will take you where you want to go! *~Michelle Segar PH.D, Behavioural Sustainability Scientist, Speaker and Bestselling Author of No Sweat: How the Simple Science of Motivation Can Bring You a Lifetime of Fitness*

Kristy has written a book that highlights the best strategies for true health and well-being. After reading, I knew that this was a book I wanted my granddaughter to read. I believe these 6 elements of health are essential to helping our young people navigate today's world. Regardless of age, this book is helpful in defining where we can improve our health to create more happiness and peace. A great treasure! *~Diane St.Jean, Client, Health Enthusiast, Mother & Grandmother*

Based on both her own experiences and her extensive education, Kristy has found an approach to health and wellness that is refreshingly straightforward. I love that she has an obvious focus on body awareness and on paying attention to the cues that your body is giving you, and then using those cues to treat and heal in an integrative manner. If you are looking for some simple practical guidance and direction with your health, this is your book! *~Kathy Leake, Owner of Straight Up Fitness & Personal Training*

I love this book! It's straightforward, authentic, and easy to read. It's jam packed with practical tools we can all use to create a healthier and more holistic lifestyle. I thoroughly appreciate Kristy's ability to intertwine research with real life stories. Such an amazing read. *~Anita Melin MA, Registered Clinical Counsellor*

Kristy has done a wonderful job at taking many factors of health and explaining them in a friendly and compassionate way. I hope this book inspires people to reach for new opportunities that will help their minds and bodies feel better. Kristy has written a book that I think everyone can benefit from reading. *~Dr. Shelby Entner, Founder & Physician at Vero Health Naturopathic Care*

Inspiring! Kristy's keen insight, combined with her client based experience makes for a most relatable journey of self exploration. This book has given me permission to accept, love, and take better care of this body I've been given. Thanks for getting me inside my head and challenging me to ditch the excuses, change my patterns, and move forward. *~Jennifer Brown, Client & Mother Extraordinaire*

This book is very well written and an outstanding resource for anyone looking to improve their health and well-being. The passion behind the personal stories as well as the client stories make it relatable, interesting, and a joy to read. Great work! *~Dominick Tousignant, Founder & President at Body Energy Club Vitamin & Supplement Store*

This book will start you down the road to a healthier and happier life. It will teach you how to create sustainable healthy habits in your body and mind; no fad diets or brutal workout regimes necessary. Kristy's writing has confidence and enthusiasm, it was a pleasure to read. This book may just change your life. *~Murphy Armstrong, Cyclist & Health Enthusiast*

Kristy has written a thoughtful and personable approach to guiding one's life into greater health. Her writing is accessible and relatable. Her 'elements' are insightful reminders for me, as I continue my lifelong practice of well-being. I love her compassionate yet very motivating approach in this important roadmap to attaining personal wellness. ~*Angelina Rosa Smedley-Kohl, Filmmaker & Librarian*

Kristy Ware has created an incredible guide on achieving optimal health. Her latest book, *Synergize Your Health: The 6 Elements for Greater Vitality and Joy,* is a wonderful culmination of her years of working with clients and developing an understanding of how true health and vitality is achieved. A must read for anyone wanting to attain ultimate wellness. ~*Janine Hannis, Educational Consultant, Health & Wellness Enthusiast*

This book was delightful to read and so applicable to everyone. Kristy's insights to the world of health and self-actualization is evidently clear. She's a true master. The vulnerability she demonstrates by sharing her own history and struggles make it so relatable. This book is a very valuable tool to everlasting change and a new perspective for anyone who can be disillusioned by the modern world. ~*Christine Poole, Client & Licensed Practical Nurse*

CONTENTS

For my family, friends, clients, and you the reader.

For every person with the courage to make changes that will lead to greater vitality and joy.

FOREWORD

It is not often you meet someone who has a permanent smile and who exudes kindness and compassion. Kristy is one of those people. I first met her when she attended a course I was teaching back in 2017. She came in with a friendly smile, kept it throughout the course and left with it too! She was a joy to teach also because of her continuous curiosity to understand why.

I believe it is this need to understand and know more that led Kristy to writing this book. She is a seeker of knowledge with a desire to live her best life and her life experiences, research and client work has allowed her to take all she has learned and share it in these pages. Not only does she want to live her best life but she wants that for you, as well. With a deep desire to serve, Kristy is driven to help others achieve their 'best life' goals.

In this book, Kristy has compiled 6 key elements for greater vitality and joy. I would hazard a guess that EVERYONE wants greater vitality and joy and would benefit from reading this book. Kristy incorporates her personal story with those of her clients, as well as evidence-based information she has gathered. She's organized it into an easy to follow book with an accompanying workbook that individuals and organizations can use to create synergy between the elements. The personal struggles she shares are a true reflection of her tenacity and spirit and are a source of inspiration for others.

As a fellow wellness enthusiast and fitness professional, I can relate with some of Kristy's struggles and enjoyed a new perspective on how to find balance again. I find personal stories very compelling as they help me connect to the writer, even when I don't know the author personally and especially powerful when I do.

Kristy's book is coming out at a perfect time - 2021. The year 2020 was one that many would like to forget but there was also a lot to learn from the challenges we faced. Health and wellness have become a priority for many who have recognized the importance of improving their health, boosting their immunity and living their best life. The 6 elements are perfectly summarized with easy to implement tips that will help so many readers transform their lives.

We live in a world with so much information and knowledge available but it can be overwhelming to know where to start. Start here with the 6 elements. This book has the power to transform and inspire many and be the catalyst to improved health and well-being.

Kim Vopni
Restorative Exercise Specialist™
Educator, and Author of *Your Pelvic Floor*

SYNERGIZE YOUR HEALTH

INTRODUCTION

This much I know for certain: life is not a straight line you follow from where you were, to where you are, to where you want to be. It's more like a forest path, scattered with fallen tree branches to step over, rocks to boulder, ditches to leap, valleys to descend, and mountains to climb. Such life experiences have the ability to bring us a greater sense of awareness and self-confidence. They can be our greatest teachers. When we are open to learning their lessons, they show us what's possible.

My life lessons, infused with those of many of my clients as well as scientific medical research, have enabled me to discover the 6 elements of health, vitality, and joy: rest, movement, connection, nutrition, mindfulness, and self-love. Each element represents a fundamental aspect of our health. When all six are synergized, they form a hexagon. They entwine to produce a joint effect greater than the effects they could achieve separately. As you read through the chapters you will see several italicized words with an asterisk (*) attached. These words are defined in the appendix at the end under 'Kristy's Health Definitions.'

Ever wonder why the hexagon is the most common shape in nature? Because it's the most mechanically stable shape there is. Hexagons can be found everywhere: in beehives, columns of lava rock, snowflakes, human cells, and turtle shells among many others. As a result of the hexagon's integrity, many man-made objects have been created following this strong geometric pattern: nuts and bolts, pencils, interlocking bricks, quilts, and soccer balls, to name a few. When strength and reliability are needed, the choice is the hexagon.

As I explain each element of the hexagon in detail in the chapters to follow, you will soon see which areas of your life could use a little more care and attention. You will understand how each element intersects with the others and how each is a part of the whole.

The elements have nothing to do with external factors and everything to do with ourselves. Each and every one of us has life experiences that lead us along our path. We are faced with adversity, triumphs, and choices at each stage in life, from childhood to the present day. Some of these choices we get to make ourselves and others feel beyond our control. I, for one, am a big believer in things happening for us, not to us. We may not know why we are facing a certain experience as we're in the midst of it, but I believe there is always something bigger at play.

As children we are constantly getting feedback from those around us to help us make sense of the world. That's what helps to shape our perspective, actions, and our decisions. Then, one day, we break free of the construct of what we thought we knew, and forge our own path with new-found information. The more I've learned to tune in into my body and mind, the simpler it's been to *synergize** my health. The 6 elements of health form a hexagon. When each functions as part of the whole, living a life with consciousness, health, and vitality is easier to achieve. When one element becomes out of alignment, the hexagon loses its integrity and balance, just as we do.

My hope is that this book helps you find and create your balance. On your own terms and in your own way. I'm here to give you the tools but it's up to you to decide how you want to use them. The things that have brought you to where you are today are neither good nor bad. They are not something you deserved, and they are not your fault. They are simply your truths. The moment we embrace our truths is the moment we are set free to live our best life. I would like to share some of mine.

IN THE BEGINNING

My mom and dad divorced when I was a year old. I don't remember a lot about those early years, just my mom and I, but what I do remember is my red, kid-sized duffle bag with the words 'Going to Grandma's' on the side. I remember packing that thing to the max with snacks, colouring books, and crayons, ready to go to my grandma's. To this day I still bring snacks in my pack even for short trips. You never know when you might get hungry! Colouring was my outlet and my most cherished pastime.

From early on, my mom became my rock, my safety net, and the person to whom I turned for everything. A few years after the divorce my mom remarried and together we moved from our urban one-bedroom apartment to a big home in the country with my step-dad. I grew up in a predominantly white, rural, conservative community in southern Ontario. I had a great childhood with lots of love and space to run, play, and get dirty.

When I was six, my sister Ashley was born. My parents were over the moon as this signified the beginning of their very 'own' family and this good feeling led to the birth of my second sibling, my brother Richard, when I was eight. This event marked a very pivotal experience and one of the most stressful times in my childhood and my family's life. My brother was born with a birth defect called spina bifida and suffered brain damage due to hydrocephalus (fluid on the brain). The severity of his conditions gave him a life expectancy of only three days. His birth was traumatic and it changed the way every member of my family viewed the world. Due to his fragile condition and high health risks, McMaster Children's Hospital in Hamilton, Ontario became my family's secondary home for almost four years. The nursing staff became our friends and when we arrived on my brother's ward each day to visit, it felt like walking onto the set of Cheers, only without the laughter and the beer.

This experience shaped my view of doctors and medicine, for which I am forever grateful. It also instilled fear and uncertainty in my life. To the doctor's astonishment and to everyone's disbelief, Richard survived multiple surgical procedures over his lifetime and even kidney failure at the age of 18. Even more miraculous – he's still with us today, more than 33 years later! As you can imagine, my brother's birth set the stage for how I viewed health, medication, stress management, the strength of family, and the true meaning of connection.

Many years ago, like many people in their early 20's, I thought I had it all figured out. I thought I knew what health was and I was living my best life. Ha. Not the case. I had no idea my perception of what it meant to live a happy, healthy lifestyle was so screwed. I used to over-exercise and under-eat. I loved the natural high exercise gave me. I used it as a way to escape and shift focus from the stress, fear, and worry in my life. But, I often used it to a fault. The food choices I made contained way too much sugar and not enough nutrients to feed my excessive exercise habits. Not a recipe for health or performance.

Mindset practice? I had no idea what that was, let alone have one. Meditation and journaling were things that 'others' did. They weren't for me and I couldn't see how they would benefit my life. At least, those were my beliefs back then. Instead, I turned to pharmaceutical medications to manage my poor digestive health and that only made me feel worse, not better. I had depression medication on refill at the local pharmacy to 'manage' my depression and anxiety. I longed to find a better way. I wasn't depressed; I was out of balance. I wanted freedom from the reliance on medication, but at the same time I felt trapped and unsure. I was far from living a healthy and happy lifestyle. I just didn't know then the things I know now, more than 20 years later.

In my mid-20's I began to explore the concepts of health and wellness beyond what I had learned from my family and my limited worldly experience. An entirely new sphere began to open up before me. Up to that point in my life all I had known was that when there was a problem with my health, I would make an appointment with the family doctor, get a prescription, take medication, and have surgery as necessary. There was no education around natural medicine, or using food to heal, or the importance of things like journaling, counselling, and meditation to address stress and anxiety, both of which played a big role in my life and sometimes still do. I don't blame anyone for what I didn't know then. In fact, all I feel is gratitude. I truly believe the path I have followed was exactly the path that was meant for me.

But, at some point, I did realize there had to be other options beyond Western Medicine and that's when I began to seek out natural healing modalities and discover practices on my own. I didn't change my ways and gain a better understanding of health overnight. Instead, my personal life experiences combined with my years of education in the fields of kinesiology, nutrition, and coaching have brought me to this point in my life, to writing this book, and sharing the elements of health with you.

Achieving overall health and well-being is about creating a balance in the way we care for the physical, emotional, and spiritual parts of ourselves. I didn't understand this concept nor its magnitude until my early 30's. After many breakdowns in my physical health and my emotional life, I began to connect the pieces of my past and understand how each event along the way led to a series of beautiful and profound breakthroughs. I had to experience the low valleys in order to reach the mountain peaks and I'm still on that journey to this day. No matter how far along the path you are, there is always room for improvement and growth.

It took years for all the pieces of the puzzle to fall into place but they have now. The 6 elements of health have been a part of me all along. I just didn't know how to tap into them before. As kids, the only coping mechanisms available are the ones that adults teach us, or, with a stroke of luck, the ones we stumble upon ourselves. Exercise became my primary outlet, second only to colouring and crafts. I lived for sports and played on every recreational team I could during elementary and high school. It was how I coped, how I celebrated, how I managed my stress - and still do.

Our life experiences are what shape us. The story we tell ourselves is what gives them power.

I have been told on many occasions by family, friends, clients, and audiences that if I could bottle up my energy and self-motivation and sell it, they would buy it! Although that in itself is not possible, what I can offer are relatable stories and simple, effective tips and tools that will make better health and greater well-being achievable for you, too. I can inspire you to take action, but the real motivation must come from within. I want to make the act of self-care possible for anyone, no matter who you are or what stage or age you're at.

Some of the things I share you may have read or heard before, but maybe this time they will really hit home. Like when someone says something to you that you've heard a few times before, then suddenly, it clicks. Maybe it's because you're in a different place in your life this time. Maybe, there's no apparent reason at all. Either way, I'm glad you're here!

Here's a little exercise I would like you to try. Grab a pencil and place each of the 6 elements in the triangle below, with the element that feels most natural and habitual to you at the top, and the one you have to work at most near the bottom. If you feel any are equal, put them side by side. This process is designed to help you rank each element of your health from 'this comes easy to me' to 'this still needs more attention'. The way you decide to rank your elements today is likely to change over time and that's totally fine.

The 6 elements of health are: *rest, movement, connection, nutrition, mindfulness*, and *self-love*.

Here's how I rank mine: How would you rank yours?

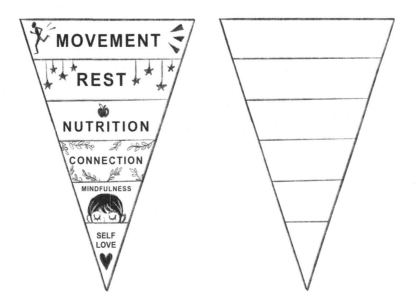

I have found this to be a very challenging but insightful exercise. It has helped me realize the areas of my health to which I give a lot of attention, and those which could use more. Maybe it will do the same for you.

We can accept life as it is, thinking we're powerless to change anything, or we can seek answers beyond what we know. We have the ability to choose what we do with our time, our energy, and our bodies. Each and every story you read in this book is true but the names of the people have been changed to protect the privacy of my clients. I designed this book to showcase my clients and my own journey to improved health, as well as to share strategies to stimulate feelings of empowerment, inspiration, and motivation in your life.

My hope is that this book helps you to reconnect with *you* – with what brings *you* joy, with what nourishes *you* – and helps bring *you* back into alignment if you've drifted off course. Each element and each chapter provides you with effective ways to synergize your health, helping you become the self-loving, well-nourished, active, and conscious individual you desire to be, one small action at a time.

My hope is that by the time you finish reading this book you don't survive in life, but thrive. It's not about doing everything perfectly, it's about making steady, positive progress. It's about committing to yourself through consistent practice and about knowing beyond a shadow of a doubt that the life you want is possible.

I'm ready. Are you?

Yours in health,

Kristy Ware

THE 6 ELEMENTS OF HEALTH

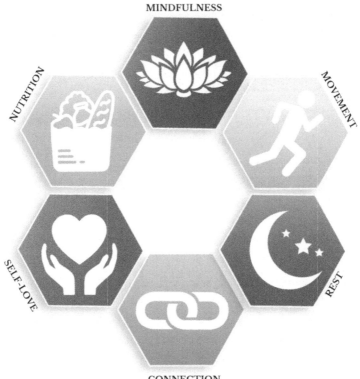

1

REST

*R*est is the first element of health. Not because it's more important than the others, but because of the enormous impact that rest, recovery, and sleep habits have on every other area of your life. Your ability to thrive is a direct reflection of your habits and routines, especially around sleep. In order to truly experience a life of well-being the first order of business is to dial in your practices around bedtime, sleeping, and waking.

The amount of sleep you need changes slightly over your lifetime. Things that make the biggest impact are age, pregnancy, previous nights of sleep deprivation, medical conditions, and the quality of your sleep. Research done by the Mayo Clinic states that in order to reach maximum productivity, immune function, and overall health, adults need between seven and nine hours of sleep each night. Living in a constant state of sleep deprivation is just as bad as oversleeping. The goal is to find the sweet spot that works for you and to create healthy habits so that getting quality rest is the norm.

Sleep patterns and routines that work for one person might not work for another. The amount of rest one needs also differs slightly from person to person. The goal is to figure out what works for your body and mind, and do it. Figuring out the sleeping and waking routine that keeps your engine happily humming along will increase your energy, patience, and concentration, while decreasing your experience of brain fog, fatigue, and food cravings.

If you're a parent, you know all too well the impact lack of sleep has on your productivity, mental energy, and will power. I recognized how much rest and recovery my body really needed after the birth of our son. I knew I valued my sleep and without a solid eight hours I felt crummy, my energy tanked, and I craved way more sugar than usual. But, like most new parents, I thought I would adapt. Boy was I wrong. Nobody can prepare you for the number of sleepless nights and sleep-deprived days you will experience when you have a newborn.

Many of my routines and habits changed drastically after our son's birth. This was due in part to the necessity of caring for him and my nursing wife, and in part because I was physically wiped out. My wife and I were up one to four times a night until our son was two years of age and started to sleep through. Even then it wasn't a given we would get eight solid, uninterrupted hours of rest.

My energy was no longer what it used to be so my physical fitness took a back seat. Instead of spending an hour a day at the gym I was doing 20-30 minute circuit-style workouts at home on the days I could muster up the stamina. Shortly after my son's birth I also became a coffee drinker to combat the exhaustion. In the end, I'm not sure how much it really helped. (Those afternoon caffeine crashes were pretty serious.)

Proper sleep hygiene repairs your cells, recharges your battery, and reorganizes your thoughts.

Something else I realized during that blissful time in new mom land was that I could no longer 'push through'. I needed to allow my body time to rest. I even started slipping away for short naps during the day while our son napped, something I was not used to doing. I had experienced enough major injuries to know that pushing through did not end well. Once I had a child, I began to value my sleep and my overall health more than ever, and I started listening even more closely to my body's needs.

Sleep is not something that you want to compromise on. While less 'conspicuous' than the other five elements, when the quality of your sleep is hindered, so are the others. Not enough sleep means that the energy you need to move your body is not there. Not enough sleep means you crave things like sugar, salt, and caffeine. It means you will lack focus, patience, and motivation. You get the picture. Creating and living with good sleep habits will have a profound effect on your entire life.

PREVENTING BURNOUT

Most of us can name someone in our lives who has experienced extreme burnout. You might have even experienced it yourself at one time or another. I know I certainly have. Back in 2007, co-founder and editor-in-chief of *The Huffington Post*, Arianna Huffington, succumbed to burnout in a big way. I share her story because her experience had such a profound effect on her life that she went on to write a book about it, *The Sleep Revolution: Transforming Your Life, One Night At A Time*. In this excellent publication, she shares her personal story as it relates to the importance of sleep, its effects on your entire life, as well as simple tips to help you get a handle on your sleep habits.

Arianna talks about her childhood and the good sleep habits she learned from her mother and how militant her mom was about sleep. In the face of Arianna's work, success, and family life, however, these lessons lost relevance. This is something many people around the globe are struggling with. There is simply 'not enough time' in the day to get everything done, so something has to give. What is that something? Yup, for most people it's their sleep.

Arianna's sleep hygiene had been sliding for years when it finally hit a breaking point. After spending several days traveling, speaking, and attending TV appearances with very little *downtime** or proper rest, she had run herself into the ground. She felt, like many, that if she wanted to be successful she needed to do it all. She was the face of her company and therefore would do whatever it took to keep things chugging along, sleep or no sleep. Not a recipe for productivity or long-term success.

Eventually, she literally dropped. She stood up from her desk to attend to something when she fainted and fell to the ground smashing the side of her face on the corner of her desk on her way to the floor. The results were a broken cheek bone, a bloody mess, and numerous visits to the doctor. Talk about burnout at its worst. The time it took for her to attend to her injury and ongoing medical appointments meant less time for her business and for her family. I love how the universe provides us with an experience to help us see what was right there all along.

The most interesting part of her experience, says Arianna, was that while she was being a superstar mom by day and a workaholic by night, she knew she was heading down a slippery slope of sleep deprivation. The signs and symptoms were all there but she dismissed them in the face of her work and family life. Like so many people, she had accepted the illusion that in order to achieve success, sleep deprivation was inevitable.

Sadly, this is how success is often portrayed by celebrities, successful business people, and by the media. If you aren't working like a dog around the clock, you will not achieve your goals. This could not be further from the truth. In order to truly thrive we must get enough quality sleep. Rather than compromise sleep, it's something to prioritize. Good sleep habits and routines are essential to a life of health and well-being.

Make choices that refresh your brain and refuel your body.

As a society, we must shift from the 'sleep is for sissies' perspective to one of respect. Instead of dismissing sleep as a time waster, view it as a time saver. Sleep deprivation and burnout are extremely detrimental to your health, decision-making, work performance, personal life, physical health, and sex life. No amount of caffeine or stimulant can replace a good night's sleep.

It all comes down to choice. You get to choose when to shut down at the end of the day. You get to choose the limits you place on your office hours. You get to decide how you spend your evenings and your spare time. By making a few, very simple decisions, you have the ability to change your entire life, as Arianna says, 'one night at a time.'

YOUR IMMUNE SYSTEM

Are you a night owl or an early bird? Does it even matter? Some people love staying up late, or heading out in the dark of night for a walk or jog. These people have lots of energy in the evening and get their most creative and inspired ideas after dark. Then we've got the other group, the early birds. These people enjoy a quiet, peaceful morning, watching the sunrise, getting their body moving right away, and wake up energized and ready to conquer the day.

As it turns out, it doesn't matter which camp you're in, the important piece is that you get enough quality rest each night. There are several scientific studies that look at how genetics play a role in our night- or day-loving fates and how our choices impact our productivity and risk for illness and injury. What scientists have found is that both the routines of your parents and your genetic make-up could be responsible. Who knew? Truth be told, no matter what time your head hits the pillow, the important piece is that you develop good bedtime and waking routines for optimal rest and *recovery**.

Sleep builds a strong immune system just like food gives us life and nourishment. What you feed your body is in direct correlation to how you are going to feel. When you eat a slew of fast food, drink too much alcohol, or eat too many sweets, your engine does not run well and you feel sluggish and depleted. The same is true about lack of sleep. You are more likely to wake each morning feeling refreshed and recharged when you get enough quality rest so your body and mind can function at their best.

Not just your external actions get affected; lack of rest compromises your internal processes as well. It's during sleep that your immune system goes to work, warding off illness, and repairing your muscles, organs, and cells. It is a huge job and not one that can be done while your body is awake warding off the ill effects of stress, poor food choices, inactivity, environmental impacts, and other demands of daily life. In fact, it's such a big job, it takes all night.

Rest and relaxation are insurance policies for your body's ecosystem.

Another interesting and related subject is the ill effect that shift work has on the body. Lots of professions have varied working hours or rotating shifts that cause changes and major disruptions to sleeping and eating patterns. As much as shift work is unavoidable for many people, it comes with a host of potential risks, including insomnia, diabetes, gastro-intestinal disturbances, and increased risk of injury or accidents. When the body does not get proper rest, it cannot function optimally.

If you've been a shift worker, you know exactly what I'm talking about. After a few night shifts, followed by a quick turn-around to days or afternoons, you feel delirious, exhausted, and 'hung-over'. The immune system becomes compromised pretty quickly and your circadian clock gets out of sync. It is important for everyone to set up good bedtime and waking routines; for shift workers, such routines are crucial.

Lack of rest penalizes you in other ways, too. You end up with a low sex drive (nobody wants that). You make poor food choices (hello sweets and deep fried carbs). You crave more coffee and caffeine (yet a caffeine overload only makes a bad situation worse). An ongoing lack of sleep can even lead to weight gain (not fair but true).

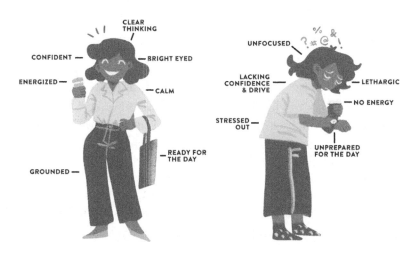

Practising beneficial bedtime routines and rituals offer the best support to your body's immune system. Simple ways to support your immune health are taking a warm Epsom salt bath before bed to help with relaxation; eating lots of fresh fruits and vegetables during the day to provide nourishment; moving your body each day through exercise; maintaining a healthy body weight for your body type; drinking alcohol in moderation (more on this in Chapter 4); not smoking; and going to bed and waking at the same time each day. By doing some of these very simple but important things, we can set ourselves up for greater overall health, better rest, and recovery.

SLEEP DEPRIVATION

The scary but sad truth is that, according to an article from the Centre for Disease Control and Prevention (CDC) in the USA, one in three adults do not get enough sleep. The CDC put out a report focused on morbidity and mortality as it relates to health. The article explains that the prevalence of healthy sleep routines varies by race/ethnicity, geographic location, the type of work people do, their educational level, and marital status. The fact that a third of people in the USA are sleep-deprived is staggering. The CDC goes on to explain how sleep deprivation has a direct correlation to rates of obesity, diabetes, high blood pressure, stroke, heart disease, and mental disturbances (for example, trouble processing information and confusion).

Without enough sleep your body and your brain do not work well together. You know what I'm talking about. You've had those days when you are much clumsier, struggle to put together a coherent sentence, and feel like you're literally dragging yourself around. We've all been there and it sucks!

I will never forget when I was 19 and almost died due to sleep deprivation. I worked with the Military Reserves part-time on weekends, while attending college during the week. Each weekend had a different focus and skill to master. One weekend we learned how to shoot a rifle at the ranges, another weekend was all about gas masks and throwing grenades. And, my least favourite weekend of the entire course and an experience I will never forget, was the three-day experience called 'managing extreme sleep deprivation in preparation for war.'

I thought of every possible excuse to get out of attending that weekend. But, I was told if I didn't, I would not pass the course and I would be expected to re-do the training. I left home on Friday morning at 5 am to head off to college. As you can imagine, that plan did not bode well for a weekend ahead without any sleep. Not a wink.

Whoever thought this was a good idea was crazy! The weekend was intense to say the least. The first 24 hours were manageable but after that I started feeling like I was hung-over. My brain was foggy and my attention and focus dissipated with each passing hour. There was no second wind. My body began running on autopilot and fumes. By day three I was stumbling around the camp like a zombie. I felt delusional and sick.

Sleep deprivation greatly affected not only my ability to think, react, and move, but also what I wanted to eat. I remember devouring junk food, chocolate bars, and any simple carbohydrate I could get my hands on. My body was crashing hard and what I needed was sleep.

The worst part of the entire experience was the drive home on Sunday evening, three days post-sleep dep. My dad had lent me his new pick-up truck as it had more space to carry all my gear, something to which he reluctantly agreed, and never did again. It was his 'baby'.

I was in no position to drive home from the camp that night. Despite being delirious, I remember how I felt that evening jumping into the truck, getting behind the wheel and hitting the highway home. It was as if I'd had a weekend bender but without the booze. I felt intoxicated and my legs seemed filled with lead.

Sleep deprivation is a feeling like no other and one you never want to experience. If you have, I feel for you.

I barely made it home that night. As I travelled at over 80 kilometres per hour along the highway, I went to change lanes. I signaled to move from the left passing lane to the right lane, but I didn't see a smaller truck in my blind spot. Suddenly a horn began blasting beside me. It was coming from the guy in the small truck I had nearly run off the road.

My hands trembled, my heart raced and I was in full on panic mode. I had nearly totaled my dad's truck and hurt someone, or worse. Luckily, the other driver was on the ball and paying attention. He drove up beside me honking and yelling, signaling me to pull over. I did so, partly because he was asking me to and partly so I could compose myself.

As you can imagine, the other driver hopped out of his vehicle and gave me a piece of his mind, which I deserved. I tried to explain myself but he was having no part of it. I was in the wrong and there was no way out. Thankfully nobody was hurt. After we parted ways I white-knuckled it all the way home where I thankfully arrived safely, crashing into my bed upon arrival.

Sleep does for your body what meditation does for your mind.

Sleep deprivation comes at a massive cost. It affects every single function in your body and your mind. According to research out of Australia, being awake for 17 to 19 hours (a typical day for most people) can have the same impact on cognitive function as a blood-alcohol level just under the legal limit for driving. Can you imagine what three days of sleep deprivation would measure? It's off the chart and gives sleep deprivation an entirely new meaning.

Looking back, a better decision would have been for me to have arranged a ride for myself. But we live and learn. Although this is an extreme example, it shows how much our bodies depend on sleep to function, and especially to focus while behind the wheel of a car. This situation could have ended very badly for me or the other driver, or both. Going 72 hours without rest was a prescription for disaster.

Skipping out on sleep is not macho or cool. Sleep deprivation causes driving fatalities and injury and illness every day. If you could do one thing today that would change your life for the better, it's placing your sleep at the top of your priority list. Create a bedtime and waking routine that supports your rest and recovery at any cost.

WAKING ROUTINES

If you didn't grow up with regular waking and bedtime routines, or your routines have changed (in not so great ways) since you became an adult, guess what? There is no time like today to create new and improved habits. As you have learned, doing so will have a massive impact on your overall health.

First, let's look at waking routines. You may never have given much thought to your alarm clock before, but you will now. Are you someone who wakes each morning naturally, to the sound of birds chirping in the yard, waves crashing the shore, or to the gentle, patient chime of a Zen clock? If you do, that's a fantastic way to go! But, most of the population wake to the buzzing of their phone beside their head, or an old school battery alarm or watch beeping rudely on the nightstand.

The way you are woken each morning is important because it sets the tone for the day ahead. The jolt of a loud buzz or beep is not the same as waves calmly rolling, animal sounds, or a simulated sunrise (or a real sunrise, depending on where you live in the world). A gentle awakening from your slumber makes for a calmer morning overall. I encourage you to think about how you want to feel each morning and how you can accomplish that. The more serene and calm our waking 'alarm', the less stress we feel as we open our eyes to the day.

Striving for perfection leads to defeat, striving for progress leads to success.

Another great way to start your day with ease and calm is to avoid hopping onto your phone upon waking. Storing it elsewhere in the house is an even better idea. Out of sight, out of mind! Your brain gets the time to wake up and process the day ahead without external sources of stress. Did you know that it takes your brain 30-60 minutes to wake up from sleep? What you do within that first hour may either set you up for success, or throw you into a negative spiral of comparisonitis, stress, anxiety, or feeling as if you're missing out. When going to bed and waking up follow relaxed, leisurely routines, your body and mind are better prepared for what lies ahead.

Snoozers take note: if you are someone who hits the snooze button five times before actually getting out of bed, you will find what I'm about to share very interesting. Sleep cycles last about 90 minutes. If you hit the snooze button then drift back into dream-land only to be jolted awake five minutes later, time and again, it causes problems for your brain. Your body begins to drift back into a sleep cycle but doesn't get to finish it.

Although it seems like a good idea, this isn't a way to get more rest — it actually does the exact opposite. Believe it not, those short snoozes will make you feel more tired and lethargic than if you got out of bed the first time your alarm went off! If you need to be out of bed by 7 am, instead of snoozing from 6:30-7, do yourself a favour, set your alarm for 7, get solid sleep for that extra 30 minutes without interruption, and then get up. You will get more rest and your body will have more energy.

You may be reading this saying to yourself, sure Kristy, that's easy for you to say, but I'm just too tired and enjoy my snooze time. What if you tried it for one week? See for yourself the difference that getting a solid 30 minutes extra ZZZ's can make in your day. You can make this transition easier if you put your alarm clock on the other side of the room. This will force you to get out of bed to shut it off when you actually need to. Once you're up, keep on moving right on into the bathroom for your morning pee, teeth brushing, and face washing. Head on into the kitchen, grab yourself a glass of H_2O – and bam, you are on a roll.

Unhurried intentional morning routines are what set you up for the day ahead. There is nothing worse than running around the house in a panic trying to get ready and feeling like you're racing the clock all day long. By banking a little extra time in the morning for self-care you are setting yourself up for a calm, grounded, and successful morning.

BEDTIME ROUTINES

Bedtime routines aren't only for kids. In fact, by committing to some very simple yet impactful routines each night (that do not involve the use of technology), you set yourself up for a better night of rest. There is a time for scrolling social media, checking emails, and playing games. Before bed is not that time.

There is a caveat here: I'm in no way trying to convince you to ditch your meditation app or the calming music on your YouTube channel that helps you unwind. What I'm asking you to consider is whether your bedtime routines are hindering or supporting your ability to get proper rest.

Research by the *National Sleep Foundation* shows that technology is seriously affecting the quality of our sleep, in three main ways:

1) Tech use suppresses our body's natural melatonin production, the hormone responsible for sleep / wake cycles. AKA, your circadian rhythms.

2) Whether you're playing games, watching a movie or sending off a few emails before bed, your brain is being stimulated and alerted by the use of a screen.

3) Keeping a phone in your bedroom interrupts your rest. The chimes, dings, screen light-ups, and buzzes coming in through the night or early morning affect the quality of your rest. Having your phone handy can also lead to poor waking habits as discussed in the previous section.

To help maximize the quality of sleep my family and I get, we have one very simple *rule**. Devices are not brought into the bedroom. They are left in the kitchen, on or near the phone charger overnight. It's a rule we've decided matters to us because it creates purposeful time for conversing, reading, stretching, foam rolling (one of my favourite things), and intimacy that doesn't happen when our eyes are attached to our phones. Believe me, banishing your phone from the bedroom will impact your life for the better.

A dark room, a quiet night, a peaceful sleep, a wakeful morning.

In every presentation I do on *self-care** I always ask the audience whether or not they go to bed with their phones on their night stand. As you might have guessed, 90% of people say, 'Yes'. You may even be one of these people. If you're not, congratulations! If you are a bedroom phone user I want to share with you some insights that might help to shift your thinking and habit around this. If your phone is the last thing you touch before bed and the first you touch upon waking, you are not setting yourself up for a calm, restful sleep or a low-stress day ahead. When you head to bed after scrolling Facebook, Instagram, checking your email or playing games, your brain is flooded with external stress (whether or not you feel it), not to mention the stimulating blue light or excitement of gaming, if this is your jam.

The evening rituals and routines you create for yourself also set you up for better sleep. Case in point: the bedtime routine we started with our son when he was three months old. It included a warm bath, followed by a board book, songs, and feed. Eventually he became conscious of the routines and what they meant. We still follow these evening routines, adjusted to his age, seven years later. What it created for his brain and body is predictability. It also allows time for him to get into a calm state and reconnect with me or my wife at the end of the day. It sets the tone for a good night's sleep.

As adults, we too need consistency in our routines to prepare our brain and body for a sound sleep. I remember back in my mid-20's when the local arena only gave the girls' hockey teams the latest and worst ice times for our games. Sometimes I wouldn't step onto the ice until 10:30 pm on a Wednesday night. Talk about messing up my sleep patterns. Games were an hour long, and by the time I got home I was hungry and wired and up way past my usual 9 pm bedtime. I was lucky if my head hit the pillow before 1 am.

Instead of getting my usual seven to eight hours of sleep, I got four to five on those nights. The next day I felt awful. I craved sweets even more than I normally did, had no energy, and my entire day felt thrown off. Since I lived for the game and my team-mates, I accepted that for those six months of the year, I would play anyways and deal with the aftermath. It wasn't ideal, but it was my choice and it was short term.

Many things may keep you up late – later than you know you should be up, or later than you want to be. No matter what that thing is, please reflect long and hard on how important it is to you. Enjoyable and fun ways to spend your evenings while still getting to bed 'on time' is the ticket to better rest. Staying up a little later on nights when you can sleep in the next day can be fun. Go for it – once in a while. But for real, long-term benefits, create solid routines around rest and give it the respect it deserves.

Something interesting happens in our bodies and minds when we head to bed and wake around the same time. We are creatures of habit and we like predictability. Aiming to go to bed by 10 pm each night (give or take 30 minutes), and to wake up at 6 am (give or take 30 minutes), sets your body clock. For you, that eight-hour window may be something else. Whatever it may be, to improve your sleeping and waking habits, find it and defend it.

Another great way to reduce stress and to get all your great ideas and plans out of your mind is to do a brain dump before bed. I like to keep a pen and notebook next to my night stand. Just before turning out the light I take a few minutes to write down the things that I want to do or focus on the following day, or ideas or insights I don't want to forget. That way I am less likely to wake up at 2 am in a panic about forgetting something important. It may not be a fool-proof sleep hack, but it's a great place to start. Brain dumping gives you peace of mind and allows you to revisit compelling ideas at a later time, *not* while your mind is preparing for sleep!

Do you love the sounds of nature like I do? Then relaxation music might help you drift off to sleep. The sounds of waves crashing the shore, birds chirping, or rain falling is very soothing and relaxing.

This one has really worked for me. There was a period of time in my life when I was struggling to fall asleep. It was very unusual. Some nights I would crash out as soon as my head hit the pillow. Other nights, I would lie awake for hours because of stress, emotional turmoil, and uncertainty. After sharing all this with my naturopathic doctor, she recommended I try a relaxation CD. In fact, she gave me the perfect one, *Rest & Relaxation* by Mont-gomery Smith. The first few nights I fell asleep close to the CD's halfway point (about 25 minutes). But after using this tool faith-fully for a week or two, my body and my mind began to associate the music with sleep. The interval before sleep fell to under five minutes, which became my norm. The music was like magic. As the time it took me to fall asleep dropped, my overall sleep quality rose.

There are several other really great ways to calm the nervous system and prepare the body for rest: reading a book; taking a warm bath; doing yoga; stretching; meditation; deep breathing; giving and receiving a massage; or spending intimate, loving time with your partner (physical or verbal).

People who use the time before bed and after waking to plan, relax, and unwind (screen-free) are better equipped to handle the unexpected. They get sick less often and are happier overall than those who don't develop these habits. I know this to be true for myself and my family. And, after coaching hundreds of people and learning about their habits, I've found it's the thing that either sets them up for success, or impedes it. Quality rest and sleep form one of the elements of health. Make it a priority and see how much better you function and feel. The best part is, the better your night routines, the better you feel upon waking. Dialing in these two small but essential habits lead to better days overall.

IN CONCLUSION

The priority you give to rest, recovery, and sleep will directly impact every other decision you make in your day. Rest, or lack thereof, has a profound impact on your physical, emotional, and mental well-being. It impacts your reaction time, your ability to lose weight, gain muscle, and function. It also has a profound effect on your productivity, how you feel, think, and move throughout your day. Lack of sleep cannot be 'made up for' by drinking more caffeine or energy drinks; life just does not work that way. Making a few small changes to your evening routines and morning rituals will set you up for success in health and all other areas of your life.

THE SUCCESS OF PROPER REST

Renee's Story

My client Renee's biggest challenge around health was her evening food choices. For her, that window of time after supper and before bed was the toughest in which to make healthy choices. She felt as though she deserved to 'celebrate' after everything she *needed* to do was done. It was the time of day when her house was quiet, and her son was in bed. She chose to reward herself with candy, sweets, or other junk food while watching TV.

I agreed that rewarding herself after a long day was indeed a great ritual. Unfortunately, the rewards she chose didn't fit with her overall health goals. What we uncovered was that food was her way to celebrate and sometimes it was an antidote to loneliness. In order to change the habit of late-night snacking (and, more importantly, her choice of snacks) we first needed to come up with a plan to help her celebrate her day in a body-positive way and better navigate her feelings of loneliness when they presented.

What Renee really wanted was to get up early each morning before her son and spend the first 30 minutes of her day exercising. She realized, however, that sugary foods eaten late in the evening did not set her up for a good night's rest or provide the energy to get out of bed in the morning. In fact, they did the exact opposite. Most nights she stayed up later than she wanted, snacking on sweets while watching TV. When her alarm went off in the morning, she woke up feeling groggy, tired, and not at all energized to start her day, let alone get up and do exercises.

Renee and I came up with several evening rituals that could serve as a reward in place of the mindless eating, while addressing her feelings around loneliness as well. Instead of eating candy she opted for frozen fruit, such as cherries or blueberries, both of which left her satisfied but eliminated the sugar high. She also drew up a list of things that she enjoyed doing and felt good to her body and mind. Things like calling a friend or family member in the evening, writing in a journal, reading a good book, stretching, doing yoga, or using her foam roller. Renee turned her evening into a time of self-care that felt like a personal reward instead of self-sabotage.

The best part of the entire process was that after Renee began changing her evening routines, she slept better and felt more energized and inspired to get out of bed in the morning. She had enough energy and time for some exercise before heading to work. To help make this new morning routine easier, she did things like laying her clothes out the night before and setting up the PVR with the yoga routine she intended to do the next morning. These simple changes proved to have massive rewards.

Once the positive evening routines were in place, getting out of bed early a few days a week became manageable, more consistent, and rewarding. By *bookending** her day, Renee was able to create a rewarding and relaxing closure to one day, and a positive start to the next. It was a win-win!

2

MOVEMENT

*O*ur bodies are designed to move and to move often. From my own personal experience and years of coaching, I believe that in order to achieve and to maintain health, we need to move every single day.

Contrary to popular belief, the terms 'exercise' and 'movement' are not interchangeable. They are synonyms but they differ in the meanings they hold and the goals they accomplish. *Exercise* is an activity that requires physical effort and places a greater demand on the body. It involves activities that are carried out in order to sustain or improve your health, fitness, sport, or skill. *Movement,* on the other hand, is a physical change in location and body position without the need to push, force, master, or gain anything. The objective of movement is simply to be in motion.

Since 2008, I have encountered many different trends in the health and fitness industry, as well as the physical concerns of the people that come to me for coaching. We are living in a world where technological advances are happening at such a fast pace. As a consequence, we're seeing more people sitting at desks for hours on end with very little reason to move. Work that was previously done by manual labour is being replaced by machines. These shifts are leading to greater instances of obesity, cardiovascular disease, diabetes, chronic aches and pains, and other physical limitations.

On the brighter side, we are slowly seeing a shift in the way offices are set up. Options are available to encourage more movement. Things like standing and 'walking' desks are becoming the norm for companies that can afford it. Movement breaks are being encouraged and walk n' talk meetings are happening more often. These are all steps in the right direction, but there is still more work to be done.

THE WORLD'S HEALTH

Recommendations for cardiovascular exercise, physical activity (PA), strength training, and flexibility vary slightly depending on the country in which you live. For people 18 and older, Health Canada and the PA Guidelines for Americans recommend at least 30 minutes of moderate-to-vigorous cardiovascular activity five days a week. If you live in places like China, Japan, or Russia, the recommendation for people between the ages of 20 and 60 is 30 minutes of exercise, every day.

Achieving that 30-minute goal should be totally doable. In fact, there are simple ways to incorporate exercise and movement into many aspects of your life, to get you moving as often as possible.

The World Health Organization (WHO) takes a global approach to the issue, offering a standard for every single person. WHO recommends adults aim for 150 minutes of moderate to vigorous exercise each week. That equates to about 21 minutes a day. This recommendation is for the maintenance of good health and does not include goals like weight loss, maintaining weight loss, or other specific fitness- or sport-related goals. To achieve a higher level of physical fitness, you might aim for 300 or more minutes each week, or 42 minutes per day and up.

Remember, though, that these numbers are just guidelines. There will always be guidelines for things in life. As their name suggests, they are meant to guide you. They are general advice and suggestions for best practices. Given that we are not exact replicas of one another, our specific needs and goals are also going to differ. In the end, you have to make the best choices you can that work for you, your lifestyle, and your health goals.

The good news is that movement comes in at least three forms, each with its own unique health benefit. Ideally, you want to find a time and place every week to incorporate each of them.

Cardiovascular exercise like walking, biking, or swimming is great for your heart, blood pressure regulation, and for prevention of stiffness, diabetes, and arthritis-related pain.

Muscle-strengthening activities, such as lifting weights, cutting and stacking firewood, and heavy or laborious jobs, build strong bones. They prevent things like falls and injuries, as well as enhance your ability to do functional, everyday tasks. They also help to support weight loss. The more muscle strengthening you do, the easier it is to lose and maintain your weight. WHO recommends that muscle strengthening occur on two or more days every week. I believe an even better goal is three to four days a week, with plenty of variety in the activities.

Flexibility and stretching is the third form of movement you want to consider in your weekly movement routines. WHO says that we should aim to stretch all our major muscle groups at least twice a week, holding each movement for up to 60 seconds. The more flexible we are, the less likely we are to develop aches, pains, stiff joints, and injuries. Flexibility can be achieved through yoga, active, passive, or dynamic movement.

Now add up the recommended time spent on each of these three forms of movement. The average person needs a total of about 60 minutes of cardiovascular, muscle-strengthening, and stretching activity each day. The actual activities you choose will depend on your interests, where you live, your health goals, and physical ability.

Now that you know what research recommends, how are you measuring up? In what ways can you improve your daily PA quota?

When Canadians were polled in 2018 about daily PA, it turns out that 34% of them thought they met the minimum standards. But according to Statistics Canada, only 18% actually did. This means that only 18-34% of people living in Canada get enough exercise each day.

Canadians are not the only ones in need of more movement. Studies also show that one in three adults living in the United States do not get enough PA each day. There is work to be done – not only for adults but for the next generations. As a society we need to find ways to include more movement in our lives and in the lives of our families. Choosing not to move your body each day has an impact on your health and every other area of your life. In my world, getting enough exercise and moving my body is non-negotiable. It's like wearing a seat belt or brushing your teeth: it's necessary and it can save your life.

MY 'GO TO'

I am one of those people who live to move. I've always had more pent-up energy than a three-year-old and function at 'mach 10' most days. I was that kid that couldn't sit still in class and loved nothing more than being active and playing outdoors. I longed for the school bell to ring and for the teacher to dismiss us for recess so I could run, jump, climb, and swing. There was something about Phys Ed class and recess that put me at ease. It took me to my happy place like nothing else ever did, or ever has.

I first stepped onto the ball field at the age of four and continued to play sports from that point onward. If my school had a team for it, I played it, right from elementary school to the end of college when I won an award for 'Outstanding Fitness Achievement'. I lived for physical activity. I could easily get lost in the game or the joy of moving my body and all the stressors of life simply dropped away, even if just for that time.

Movement has been, and always will be, my 'medicine' of choice. It's my go-to when I'm happy, sad, stressed, overwhelmed, angry, scared, or any other emotion. It's one of the only things that has consistently brought me back into balance and given me a sense of contentment. It's when I get my most inspiring hits and my greatest ideas. It's what brings me up when I am down and what helps me rise even higher when I'm already feeling on top. Something as simple as playing soccer with my son or a walk around the block has the potential to change everything.

Although movement comes easily to me, not everything has. For most of my childhood and even into my adult life, I never considered myself a good reader. As a kid I enjoyed picture books and although I could read (slowly) I found no joy in it. I disliked book reports because they forced me to read (or to ask my friends what the book was about). Even more, I feared being singled out in class and asked to read aloud. It made my heart race and my palms sweat. I never gravitated towards reading, and therefore never built a solid foundation from which to do it. For over 25 years I had the belief and carried the story that I was not a good reader. While I'm not proud of it, I can honestly say that I never read a single book cover-to-cover until I was 29.

The point of my story is that not everything comes easy to everyone. We all have to work at something. We also have to explore our options until we find an activity, book, or hobby that we thoroughly enjoy. Some of us carry stories from our past about gym class or exercise that have dragged on for years and may no longer be true. Or if they are still true, we do have the ability to change them now.

It's easy to believe that the way things are right now is how things will always be. But guess what? You can choose something different. You can shift and reframe the story if you want to. If exercise has never felt enjoyable, only you can make the decision to change that – to find the kind of movement that you find enjoyable, and then do it!

BUST THROUGH WHAT HOLDS YOU BACK

For a multitude of reasons, people struggle to enjoy movement. Sometimes it stems from childhood. It's possible that as a kid you were told that you were not good at sports, or you always got picked last for team games. These experiences are etched in your brain. They have molded the person you are today and you still fear you are not good enough, and that you never will be.

I've heard more stories than I would like about people having negative experiences at school with teachers or coaches. These interactions have tainted their idea of exercise and negatively affected their enjoyment of it. Being singled out by a teacher in front of your classmates for your lack of skill or endurance or being pushed by the coach beyond what is enjoyable and fun can set you up for failure and overall negativity towards PA.

Another reason so many people struggle to find enjoyment in movement is the excess body weight they carry. As of 2007, Statistics Canada has deemed obesity to be a global phenomenon. Roughly 60% of adults in Canada and 69% in the United States are considered overweight or obese. These numbers are staggering and are climbing as time goes by. Living with a weight concern is a huge barrier to movement and a source of stress and embarrassment. Many adults who carry extra weight were overweight as children. This proves that healthy eating and good food choices start at home.

In fact, WHO identifies childhood obesity as one of the most challenging public health concerns of the 21st century. While the problem is global, it is highest in North America. Children who are overweight or obese are far more likely to stay that way into adulthood and are at great risk of developing non-communicable ailments, like diabetes and cardiovascular disease. Just writing this makes me sad. I'm a parent and I want nothing more than to set my son up for success. I want him to have the best nutrition and lifestyle I can provide. I want him to benefit from the impact food and movement will have on his entire life. I wish the same for all kids.

The truth is, children are mainly educated, fed, and 'cared for' by people older than them. The parental figure in their lives or the one buying the groceries gets to choose what food is brought into the home or eaten at a restaurant. The home is where health or illness begins. The rise in childhood obesity can be traced back to two factors: first, the increased intake of highly processed fat and sugar-laden foods that are low in vitamins, minerals, and other essential nutrients; and second, the trend for kids to spend more time sitting and less time physically active than ever before.

Some people are quick to blame genetic factors for this situation. Although genetics do play a role in weight management and body composition, studies show that what we eat and how we care for our bodies have a vast impact on our weight and overall fitness. Just because family members are overweight does not mean you have to follow suit. Changing your habits around food choices and exercise will change your body. Finding a starting point is often the hardest part. But when you take action on one thing, you gain momentum and motivation to take action on another thing, and then on another - that is when you really start to make changes.

Make choices today that your body will thank you for tomorrow.

Just as being overweight can keep a person from enjoying movement, so can being thin, lanky, clumsy, or uncoordinated. Becoming good at movement (like anything in life) is going to take practice – doing something over and over again. If persistence is not your strong point, find a group, class, or activity where the goal is fun, laughter, and connection, not competition. If that's too public for you, try a solo activity like skiing, walking, or swimming. Then it doesn't matter whether or not you're good at it – if you love it, it's worthwhile.

There are many excuses people have that can block them from exploring movement and finding joy in it. These excuses may not be based in fact, but having been repeated story for so long, people have come to believe them anyway. And that belief is what gives these stories energy and ensures that nothing will change.

That's why I spent so little time reading books throughout my youth. I blocked it. I didn't believe I was a 'reader'. Boy, am I glad I changed that story. Regardless of the story you tell yourself, I am here to say it's possible to change it. It's possible to find enjoyment in all aspects of life, including PA, regardless of your past experiences or present situation. What it comes down to is finding the PA that's the right fit for you. If you have not found it yet, keep trying until you do!

DITCH THE EXCUSES

Humans are really good at coming up with *excuses**. Excuses are 'good reasons' that justify or defend why we did or did not or cannot do something. They are a way to make ourselves feel better, at least in the short term. Take a look at the list of reasons you might use to 'excuse yourself' from moving your body. The moment you shift your thoughts is the moment you can change your actions.

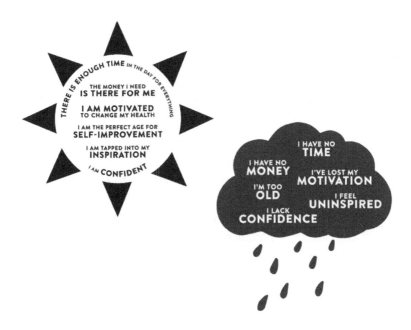

I have no time.

I hear this one all the time. Pun intended. 'I'm just too busy' to find the time for movement. Guess what? Every one of us gets 24 hours every day. It's what you choose to do with that time that's the game changer. My busy life already leaves little time for me, you say, and that may be true, but only to an extent. You are in charge of how you spend your day, which activities you choose to do, which things you make a priority, what you schedule into your calendar – and how creative you get in order to carve out the time to move your body. Movement doesn't have to take up a big chunk of time. Ten minutes at three points in the day to walk around the block or do a few squats, lunges, or push-ups will go a long way.

I have no money.

This excuse is simply not true. Most people own a pair of decent running or walking shoes and this makes moving super simple. It does not need to break the bank. Things like walking, jogging, and swimming (if you live near a lake or safe oceanfront) are great ways to increase your heart rate, your metabolism, and improve your mood. Exercises that require no special equipment, known as body-weight exercises, can be done in the comfort of your home. Money should not be a barrier to staying fit and strong. Get creative, work with what you have, and you will be surprised at how good you will feel.

I've lost my motivation.

I admit, this is a tricky one, even for me. Motivation is our general desire and willingness to do something. Some people have more personal motivation than others. I have never been challenged or paralyzed by lack of motivation, but lots of people are. Despite the variation I see from one person to another, I believe that like anything, motivation can be learned with practice and encouragement.

My client Kate (I'll share her story at the end of this chapter) admitted to me on our consultation call that she lacked motivation to strengthen and stretch her body. But she also shared that she longed to get back into downhill skiing, something she loved, without pain and discomfort. She had the self-awareness that her habits had to change but she knew she could not commit to those changes alone. After years of suffering, she dug deep to find the motivation to call me. She knew she had to commit to showing up each week (a brand new experience in her world). Within a few months of committing to herself, she saw a change in her body for the better. We are still working together over two years later and I know for a fact that motivation is what brought her to me, and motivation is what has kept her going.

**Excuses hold you back
from becoming the healthiest
and happiest version of yourself.**

I'm too old or it's too late.

Blake was in his 60's and had spent his entire working career as a baker at a big chain grocer. He had baked bread almost every day for 30 years straight. That's a lot of bread! Given there wasn't much variety in his tasks at work, his hips, low back, and pelvis had become inflexible and his posture was compromised as a result.

Blake had never stepped foot in a gym and didn't consider himself at all athletic. When his registered massage therapist referred him to my Core Confidence and Conditioning class, he could have easily refused. It was way out of his comfort zone, he was close to retirement, and he felt some apprehension. But, because his therapist recommended the class, he gave it a shot.

The first few months were challenging. He struggled to find his balance. His core was weak while his body lacked flexibility. During bent-over exercises, he could only reach down as far as his knees. He had a desire to touch his toes, something he had never ever done before. He set a goal and worked at it. Within one year of attending classes, and focusing on elongation and proper movement patterns, Blake touched his toes! It was a glorious day.

For some, this may seem basic. But for others, simply moving better means a better quality of life. That is what happens when you ditch the excuses and set your body in motion. Blake and I continue to coach privately to this day, and together, we have been setting and achieving goals ever since. He's proud to say he can now shoulder check while driving with much more flexibility and ease. He's standing taller, feeling stronger, and moving better than he ever has before. It's never too late to get started.

We all have something that motivates us. Some people are motivated by internal factors, others by external factors, and some a combo of both. Once you figure out what motivates you, it will be easier to build consistency. When you commit to yourself, your success is inevitable.

I lack confidence.

For those of you who are dealing with an injury or who have steered clear of exercise and fitness for one reason or another, getting back on track can feel daunting or even scary. You may well struggle to find the confidence to do anything. In this situation, my best piece of advice is to take the first step. That might mean walking for five minutes a day, stretching each evening before bed, or using your lunch break for power walks with a colleague.

Or, you could do something even braver, like hire a coach, a physical therapist, or fitness expert who specializes in what you need most. Hiring someone will hold you accountable; it will provide you with professional guidance, care, and support to go from where you are right now to where you want to be. The moment you take your health into your own hands is the moment you will begin to regain your confidence.

I lack interest.

Have you ever thought you would dislike something (could be food, a game, or a sport) but when you tried it, you actually enjoyed it a lot? That's the approach I like to use when coaching people. I want them to find that thing that interests them most. Not the thing I like, or the thing I think they 'should' do, but the thing in which they find joy. You will never know what you like until you try it!

What may seem like a lack of interest in movement could well be a sign that you simply don't know what excites you. It's easier to put up a wall or close yourself off than to try something unknown to you. It may feel safer, but in reality, what's at risk is your opportunity to thoroughly enjoy something entirely new. (More about this in the next section, 'Find Your Jam'.)

You may have many reasons for making excuses not to move. Yet I'm sure if you made some time to create a short list of the pros and then cons, you would discover that your reasons are not based in truth. I challenge you to really look at what's holding you back from taking better care of your body and yourself.

To make any significant change you first must figure out what motivates you to do what you do. It might be sheer desire, money, shopping, vanity, or vacations. It could be a feeling, like strength, confidence, sexiness, or less aches and pains. It might even be that you want to look better in a swimsuit. Whatever it is, push aside those excuses, grab hold of that thing that lights you up, that pushes you to get off the couch or step away from your device and make it happen. You deserve it.

FIND YOUR JAM

Do you know which movement is the best type for you? Is it walking, stretching, or weight training? Is it team sports or solo sports? The truth is, no form of movement is best for every person. The best one to do is the one that you love— and will do often. I like to use the equation, 'doing what you love + consistency = progress + results.'

The good news is that anyone has the ability to change at any time. You do not need permission to change an old pattern or way of seeing yourself. You get to decide. Just as I decided that I wanted to change when I met my future wife (a very prolific reader and intellectual). Until that time I was closed off to the idea of reading and avoided it at all costs. I put up a wall around the idea. I confined myself, my abilities, and my interests instead of being open and continuing to try and explore new things.

The best form of movement you can do is the thing you are going to stick with.

Suddenly I had a 'light bulb' moment. I found myself wanting to try something new that had not come easy to me and that I never thought I 'could' enjoy. With some encouragement and good recommendations, my wife helped me find a love of reading. I didn't care how long it took me to finish each and every chapter. Speed reading wasn't the point. Writing a report for my prof wasn't the point. Forcing myself to do something because someone else said I had to – that was not the point, either. I made up my mind to do it because I wanted to and because it felt good. Years later I marveled at the number of books I had read, enjoyed, and grown from, and felt proud of myself. Now I can't believe that I've written a book!

That is the feeling you should get from moving your body. Move in a way that feels good. Doing something because someone else has said you 'should' do it will not fuel you over the long term. Doing something because you feel deep down in your core that it will make you happier is the best fuel you can have. It comes from within. It's an internal desire to do something for yourself and do it consistently.

Finding a love for anything, be it playing a sport, biking, hiking, playing an instrument, painting, or reading, takes an openness and willingness to break through any limiting thoughts about yourself plus the genuine interest to make it a part of your life. There are certain parts of our lives in which we have little to no choice, like the community in which we grew up, the elementary school we attended, or the experiences and interests that others impose on us as children. The list goes on. But when we get to choose how we react, we react and move beyond those experiences. We get to decide the path we want to take in life and that includes choosing to move our bodies in ways that light us up.

I hope this leaves you inspired by the chance to choose a different life path, one in which movement brings you joy. Remember that we get to live with our choices, which means that it's best to make them with care as well as enthusiasm. This next section is about some lousy choices that I made around movement. It's also about how even my resulting 'mishaps' can be viewed as a source of invaluable truth about life and myself.

MISHAPS GIVE FEEDBACK

Mishap #1

I crossed the finish line as the big, red digital clock filed my bib number and time at 1 hour and 52 minutes. Even as I share this story with you I cannot believe I ran for 1 hour and 52 minutes without stopping. Who does that? I was 20 years old and thought I was invincible. I overdid it with most physical activities back then as if I had something to prove. ('To prove something' is a horrible reason to run 30 kilometres around the bay in Hamilton. Just saying.)

Only a few months before I had joined a long-distance running club. I did it as a way to relieve stress and meet new people. Up until then I had only been training to run up to five kilometres because I was preparing for the police department's physical endurance test. To pass that test, someone of my age and gender had to complete a 2.4 kilometre run in under 13 minutes and 26 seconds. I had that dialed and was not worried in the least about passing. In hindsight, I should have just stopped there. My only goal was to pass the police test – not to become an Olympic athlete!

Within less than two months of joining the club I went from running five kilometres to running 30. There was no "Couch to 30KM" in those days. Nobody thought about putting me on a slow, progressive plan to help build up my body, endurance, and strength. Instead, I pushed my body beyond what it could handle.

As I crossed the finish line of that 30 kilometre road race, I feared it was likely one of my last. The pain I felt in my right knee was debilitating. I had done too much too fast and my body had rebelled. So, at the age of 20, my two-month affair with the world of long-distance running came to an abrupt end. An MRI revealed that my meniscus was bulging into the boney area between my knee joint. It swelled and was especially painful when doing things like running as every impact pinched my meniscus. If I didn't stop running, the doc advised, I might not be able to enjoy all the other sports and activities that I loved. It was a sad day. But the lessons it taught have remained with me to this day.

During that time of physical breakdown I learned three very important things:

1. Slow progressive exercise programs are the best. Too hard, too fast just leads to injury.
2. Listen to your body and never push through pain. Constantly pushing beyond what your body is capable of will lead to physical breakdown.
3. Put aside your pride and consider the long-term implications of your actions. The only person to whom you have to answer is yourself. No matter what decision you make or actions you take, keep this in mind.

Mishap #2

My second major injury happened only a few years after my first. I will never forget that frigid winter day back in 2001 when I bundled up to brave the elements, threw on my rollerblades, and popped a Melissa Etheridge CD into my Sony Discman. It was the perfect way to prepare for my upcoming hockey tournament.

At some point during my training, while skating backwards, a twig or a stone got caught in my wheel. Oh, I forgot to mention – I was not wearing a helmet. All I recall is waking up to the sunshine glimmering through the bare tree branches above as they clacked together. The wind coming off the lake was high that day. The whole experience felt like something out of a movie.

I was confused as to why I was laying on the ground. I made an attempt to sit up but a woman yelled from a distance telling me that I should stay put and that an ambulance was on its way. Moments after that short interaction an ambulance pulled up to take me to the hospital.

The result? A third-degree concussion. The most severe blow to the head a person can experience. To the doctor's surprise, the CT scan showed no broken bones and no internal bleeding. It was a miracle. My guardian angel was watching out for me that day.

That injury left me with major vertigo and headaches on and off for several years. To everyone's surprise, the accident's only lasting repercussion was its effect on my sense of smell and taste. Given I work in an industry encouraging people to sweat, losing part of my sense of smell is not all bad. It could have been much worse and for that I am thankful.

Once again, there were three big life lessons I learned in that time of breakdown:

1. For goodness sake, wear a helmet. It's way cooler than a head injury and helmets nowadays are super funky!
2. Let someone know where you are. If it wasn't for that lady who was out walking, I could have laid on the cold hard pavement for hours. It was minus temps and that trail was almost desolate that day.
3. We are not invincible, despite what we want to believe. Our bodies are fragile and injuries of this magnitude don't just go away. They are with you for life. Be kind to your body and protect the heck out of it.

Mishap #3

My third life-altering injury happened in 2011. I was on summer break between the first and second year of my kinesiology program. I felt like I was at one of the fittest points in my life. I weight-trained five days a week, played softball, biked every day, and did a ton of sit-ups and crunches to stay strong.

I went to bed one night and woke the next morning with my back in crippling pain. As I hobbled from the bedroom to the bathroom my mind reeled to make sense of what I had done. I suffered the rest of that summer without any answers as to why my back was causing me such grief. I began my second year of college dragging a wheeled backpack to the train station each morning. Yes. A backpack on wheels, like the ones you see elderly people using when grocery shopping.

I felt defeated. I felt as if my body had failed me. Those long depressing months challenged me physically, mentally, and emotionally. What if I never walked again without pain? What if I ended up with permanent nerve damage? What the heck had caused this? I had so many questions that were, up to that point, unanswered.

Searing pain radiated from my low back and shot down into my left leg. I wanted it to stop and I wanted answers. I am a solution-oriented person and I wanted to fix it. It wasn't until Christmas, six months into that crazy journey, that I finally had a diagnosis for my horrendous back pain: two slipped or bulging discs at my L4 and L5 vertebrae that were pinching my sciatic nerve. I am not sure if having a diagnosis made my situation easier or if it just gave me a new perspective and a focus.

I took this new-found knowledge and began researching why this type of thing happens in the first place, and how to manage the pain, naturally. I wanted answers to what had caused the discs to slip in the first place. But ultimately, I wanted to know what I needed to do to heal from this awful experience.

So, what do we do in the 21st century when we need answers? Head over to Facebook, of course! I shared a post asking for advice and suggestions about how to heal slipped discs. Lots of friends and family sympathized with me and sent 'love and healing' my way. One comment changed my life, however.

Within days a good friend dropped her inversion table off at my doorstep and I began using it. If you are unfamiliar with an inversion table, it looks like a freaky S&M contraption. I brought it in, set it up and began using it immediately. I was done with medication and 'waiting it out'. I needed relief and I needed it fast. Within weeks of using that table I started to feel better. I increased the time and the angle of inversion as the months went on. In conjunction with stretching, core strengthening, and mindset work, I began to heal.

I was back playing softball the following summer, having regained more than 90% of my strength and stamina. What initially appeared to be a weak back or repetitive-strain injury actually turned out to be the result of a weak core and pelvic floor.

The very foundation of my body was weak and unable to withstand the amount of physical exertion I was asking of it.

Not long after those two very intense and trying years, I decided I wanted to specialize in core rehabilitation. I wanted to help myself recover and heal, and I also wanted to help others do the same.

The lessons from my back injury were:

1. Too hard too often = breakdown. The fact that I could strength train five days a week, play two games of softball, and ride my bike everyday for at least an hour didn't mean I needed to.
2. Sit-ups and crunches do not build core strength. Sure, defined abs look nice but core strength is something you build from the inside out. No amount of crunches and sit-ups can compete with very specific core conditioning.
3. Rest and recovery are as important as training. Rest lets the body repair, recover, rebuild, and prepare for the next training day.

If you reflect on each physical ailment or breakdown you've experienced, I'm sure you will find that it has a life lesson for you.

Learn from those lessons and move forward with your new-found knowledge. Oh, and have fun while you're at it! Life is all about adventure.

Tune into your body's messages. Ignoring them will make them louder and more fierce.

PICK YOUR PLEASURE

Having checked out the impact that choices can have in and on our lives, let's dial things back a bit. When it comes to movement, choice can be the difference between misery and pure pleasure. Like Michelle Segar shares in her book *No Sweat*, separating movement into two streams, 'structured' and 'unstructured' lends itself to more movement options. Making movement a bigger part of your life is as simple as picking the stream that pleases you most. Regardless of the way you choose to move, the end result is equally rewarding. You're stronger, healthier, and happier.

Structured movement refers to things like a 60-minute fitness class, an appointment with your fitness trainer, a softball game, soccer match, hockey practice, or scheduled walking date with a friend at lunch. All these activities are things you schedule and are done for a specific time period and with a goal in mind.

Unstructured movement, on the other hand, is everything in daily life that involves movement without a rigid time frame. Things like tending to your garden, biking to work, walking up the stairs instead of the elevator, shoveling snow, playing with your kids or grandkids, or doing household chores. These are things we do because they need to be done, and not because we have scheduled them in. Choosing unstructured movement could simply mean weaving more movement into what you normally have to do

anyway, like choosing to walk, bike, or take transit from point A to point B, instead of driving.

I have to say that a lot of people don't take unstructured movement seriously. As a result, they get down on themselves. To be healthy, active, strong, and fit, they figure, you have to be a 'jock' and go to the gym five days a week. I think that's why for so many people 'movement' becomes a burden, instead of a pleasurable part of being alive and vibrant. They overlook the impact that simply moving more often and sitting less often will have on their lives.

FIND OPPORTUNITIES TO MOVE

No Sweat was one of my favourite books of 2019. In it, Segar introduces an acronym that she and her clients came up with: OTM, meaning Opportunities to Move. It drives home the idea that we each can find motivation, and in turn better health, by simply creating more opportunities for movement throughout the day.

Segar's philosophy is on point with my own thoughts and feelings around movement and motivation. Since 2008 and starting my career in the health and fitness industry, I have seen a lot of variety in what motivates people to move. I've also seen that it is possible to find that motivation, no matter who you are, how old you are, or your life circumstances. The first step is to change your thinking around movement and what it means to you. The second step is to discover what you enjoy doing, and the third step, is to do it - often!

Segar also explores the idea that movement is a gift and that the opportunities to give yourself that gift are everywhere. Even more important, by viewing movement as a gift, you can change your mindset. Instead of a chore you have to push yourself to do, movement becomes a part of the day you look forward to, just like sleep and good food. By changing your perspective on movement, you change your motivation for doing it.

Why not give yourself the gift of more flexibility, better endurance, less pain and discomfort, more strength, and more importantly, a better state of mind – simply by moving?

We make hundreds of choices and decisions each and every day. The choices that you make have the capacity to build momentum and propel you forward, but only if you follow up on these choices with action. Nothing can change unless you make the commitment to put one foot in front of the other and never give up. I hear my dad's voice telling me, 'It's when you stop moving that you die.' As morbid as this may sound, there is a lot of truth to it.

Historically, OTM's were never in short supply. A day in the lives of our grandparents or great-grandparents looked very different from ours in the 21st century. Although many advances and inventions have benefited us, many have also hindered our necessity to move. It's hard to imagine that every detail of every day once had to be taken care of by 'someone' not 'something'. Life has been made easy by things like washing machines, dryers, dishwashers, TV remotes, and of course, the mobile phone. Each of these has helped us live better lives, while also reducing the number of our daily OTM's.

Several years into my fitness coaching career, I realized that many of the clients who wanted my support to gain strength, rehab, lose weight, and improve their health did so simply as a means to an end. They came to me with the mindset that once they reached their goal, they were done. End of story. They had a definitive end-date in mind, like a wedding or conception. Once that life event passed, they often fell back into old habits and routines.

There is nothing at all wrong with wanting to look and feel your best on your wedding day. But what if you decided that you were going to make a lifestyle change? What if you decided to make choices that would improve the longevity and vitality of your life, instead of focusing on a one-off? This would change the game you play and how long you play it. With any luck, it would change how you view movement and the choices you make each day.

PHYSICAL PHILOSOPHIES TO LIVE BY

After three major injuries and many minor ones, the point came when I realized that I could not continue pushing my body beyond its limits. I needed a more gentle approach that included stretching, yoga, and walks for pleasure, not purpose. Instead of pushing so hard, I started incorporating daily relaxation exercises into my routine. Interestingly enough, it was exactly what my body needed.

That is how 'physical philosophies to live by' was born. They are certain parameters that I needed to place in my life in order to create better physical health.

The first philosophy is what I like to call the 50/50 rule. If I planned on 40 minutes of movement in my day, I allowed myself to do what I loved 50% of that time; the other half of my time and attention I focused on what I knew my body needed. For you that could mean dancing, skating, playing sports, yoga, walking, or doing anything that lifts you up and makes you feel your best, 50% of the time. The other 50% could be spent doing those rehab exercises for that old shoulder injury, doing some basic core strengthening to help with your back pain, or doing ten minutes of yoga alongside your strength routine to keep you limber and strong. By spending 50% on what you need, you can spend the other 50% on what you love so much better!

It's not about how much you do, it's about the quality of what you do.

43

The second physical philosophy took shape after I became a parent. Regardless of how much time you have, do it anyways, because something is always better than nothing. If you have children you understand how little time is left in the day for yourself and your self-care. Even if you don't have kids, stuff happens!

If you're going to be late for a class, a game, or a planned movement date, go anyways! If you leave the office late; there's a car accident on the highway; your kid spilled milk on the floor just as you were leaving them with the sitter, go anyways!

Small annoyances can happen anytime and can easily change your plans and derail your day. It will happen. Going anyways means you'll be ten minutes late – but you still get 50 minutes of movement. It's still better than not going at all. Previous to becoming a parent, I felt that I needed 60 minutes or more of structured time to work out each day or else it wasn't worth it. I was so used to carving out that time each day without fail.

Now, I make the best of the time I do have and let go of unrealistic expectations. Once I shifted my thinking to make the most of the time that I *did have* to work out, instead of writing it off as 'not enough', everything changed. It's very easy to fall into the 'it's not worth it' mindset if you have less time than you would like or are used to. If you are used to 60 minutes and now you find yourself in a situation where you only have 20, it can feel like a waste. Take it from me, a gym junkie, it feels better to do something for 20 minutes, than doing nothing at all. That 60-minute mark had simply been a mind game that I was no longer willing to play.

When you make the choice to take every opportunity that arises as a way to move more, it becomes a reward for your body and mind. For me, those small, 20-minute blocks were and continue to be my saving grace. They add up over the course of the day. Before you know it, you have given yourself the gift of feeling great many times, instead of feeling frustrated or sluggish because you didn't.

The third physical philosophy I adopted and live by is building basic movement into my everyday life. Things like walking or biking to work. Taking the bus instead of driving, and getting off a few blocks early to walk to my destination. Parking at the back of the grocery store lot and walking further to get to the doors. Taking the stairs instead of the elevator. *Anything* that encourages more movement and that easily integrates into your lifestyle is key. There are lots of ways to move in natural and simple ways that do not require any fancy equipment or money. Get creative and see how many more times you can move than you ever thought possible.

External rules govern your conduct, but internal philosophies define your life.

You want to know one of the fastest ways to get yourself out of a slump? Get outside and walk around the block. In as little as five minutes you have the ability to change how you feel. I dare you to do it. Go. Now. I'll still be here when you get back.

Small actions like this will improve your mood, they cost nothing at all, and can be done virtually anywhere, anytime. When we move our bodies, regardless of how we move them, we not only raise our serotonin (happy hormone) but we also increase blood flow to our brains, improve our mental clarity, and decrease pain and discomfort. Do you really need any more reasons to get moving?

45

IN CONCLUSION

Unlike baseball caps and finger gloves, there is no one-size-fits-all when it comes to finding enjoyment in movement. The easiest way to improve your physical fitness is to find something you enjoy, and do it often. Focus your energy on quality not quantity, and on 'I can' rather than 'I should'. And remember, excuses can get in the way of doing all kinds of things, but they don't have to. Find what motivates you to do what you do, grab hold of that feeling you want to create, and take the next right step. Changes to physical fitness take time and patience but the mental, physical, and emotional payoff are worth it. Physical activity creates stronger bodies, healthier minds, and more joyful lives.

THE SUCCESS OF CONSISTENT MOVEMENT

Kate's Story

From the moment Kate and I spoke on the phone for her consultation I knew coaching her was going to be fun, but would also come with some challenges. One of the first things she admitted to me was that she was unmotivated to do things on her own but had goals she had been longing to achieve for years.

The sad part was that her work as an anesthesiologist was causing her aches and pains almost daily. Between lifting patients who were under anesthetic, doing medical charting, and other tasks at a desk ergonomically inappropriate for her body type, her body was rebelling and crying out for help. Combine that with erratic work hours including shift work, Kate was having a hard time scheduling consistent activity into her life. Basically, she was living in plain-old survival mode. She had not been active in several years but knew she needed to change that.

My first plan of action was to help her reduce her daily neck, knee, and sacroiliac (the joint at the base of your spine) pain. It was going to require some specific exercises on my part and some dedication on her part. Another long-time goal of Kate's was to get back into downhill skiing, biking, and simply feeling stronger in her body. She really wanted to return to the activities she had done years previous but lacked the strength and fitness level to do so now. She knew she needed professional support and guidance to get back into PA, and to remain there.

Kate and I have been working together ever since. It's been over two years and it's been such a positive journey. She arrives at each session happy and ready to go regardless of how tired she is or how much discomfort she's feeling. Although she rarely complains about the difficulty of the exercise routines I put her through, she does shoot me obvious looks of disapproval and sarcastic digs when I ask her to do things she really doesn't like.

Planks and squats are her faves … to disapprove of, that is. I don't know if she really 'enjoys' the exercises we do together at our weekly session, but she knows that it leads her to doing other fun and more exciting things. So to her, that's worth it.

That said, you can imagine the amount of creativity it takes to get Kate to do the things I know she needs. My sense of humour combined with my high level of creativity works wonders! Kate can do all sorts of planks, squats, and other beneficial exercises and most times doesn't even realize it, until she's doing it! And, the best part is that it's not taking her hours in the gym to accomplish her goals.

Last winter Kate shot me a text that read, and I quote, "So…turns out squats work. I haven't had any knee problems with my ski days and today I was skiing moguls! I've had to ice my knees after every ski day for the past 15 years. You're da bomb!"

The moral here is that when you do the things you need to do, you are far more capable of doing the things you love. Without giving strength training a try, Kate may never have experienced the improvements in her mobility and strength, and a reduction in her pain.

Regardless of whether or not she ever viewed herself as a 'gym person' or if she even likes 'strength training', Kate recognizes the benefit of it and it has changed her life. Her dedication to showing up for herself each week and putting in the work has paid off. Now she's skiing moguls (the bumpy ski hills that require good balance, coordination, and strength) pain-free! She and her husband are planning a trip that involves a bike tour. She experiences fewer flare-ups in her body and she has more fun in her life. She's become not only a client, but a friend, and I couldn't be more proud.

3

CONNECTION

*A*s you will discover throughout this chapter, the way you create connection in your life has a direct correlation to your health. Connection has three subcategories to explore: connection to yourself, to others, and to the world around you. Your ability to develop healthy relationships and a strong feeling of connection to mother earth starts with you. Self-connection is a state of being where you regularly tune into your emotions, your spiritual and physical needs, and your intuition. It's having a strong internal compass and living with a sense of fulfillment. This lends itself to creating greater confidence and joy in all areas of your life.

Humans have an innate need to belong, fit in, gather in groups, and feel part of something. The more opportunities we can create to fulfill the need for connection with others, the happier life will be.

In May of 2020 I ran a corporate group health program for a team of administrators. There were 30 individuals on staff. One of them, Miles, had a real 'go getter' personality and put 110% of his energy into every task. During one of our weekly coaching calls, he had a very insightful experience.

Until that point, Miles had never realized that his 'matter of fact' personality was getting in the way of his ability to slow down, offer pleasantries, and connect socially with his co-workers. He realized that he had been living in a state of 'it's all business' for many years, without ever seeing that as a 'problem' or as something worth changing.

What we uncovered was that his way of thinking and acting was a double-edged sword. It might be good for something like satisfying his work ethic, but not for other things, like building company morale and a more collegial workplace. He explained that he got so caught up in a task and in doing it well that he didn't connect with the humans who were helping him along the way.

I reminded him that it was OK; we all make mistakes or do things we are not proud of. I also reminded him that having grown more self-aware, he could implement change at any time. He saw where he was 'going wrong' and acknowledged the path to self-improvement. With my guidance, he also envisioned what needed to happen next. Some very small changes would improve the relationship he had with his team and with himself in return.

In the weeks to follow, he began to make a conscious effort to connect with others in his department. He began to speak more kindly, and even compliment other people's efforts. He expressed his embarrassment for not doing so earlier. He was so caught up in the work, he had lost something really important: the social connection to his co-workers.

Several weeks later, Miles shared with me that a few of his senior colleagues had pulled him aside and complimented him on how he had changed and how he had become much more open and supportive in the office. His efforts were being noticed and it felt good. This proved to be a considerable breakthrough for Miles, both at work and at home. Something as simple as stepping back and thinking before acting brought him the connection he needed. It also made his work environment and external relationships that much stronger and more enjoyable.

It can be so easy to coast through your day without stopping to think about what others around you may be feeling or thinking or how your actions and words may be affecting them. Taking the time to connect with people will help bring you back to the present, strengthen your relationships, build trust, and remind you to live as a 'human being' not as a 'human doing'. Unlike robots, we need to feel supported, valued, and loved. Genuinely connecting with another person can be the difference between a good day and a great day. Social connection is one of the 6 elements of health.

ESTABLISHING BOUNDARIES

It was 2016 and my wife and I had a dream and vision for our future. We wanted something more for our lives than a two-hour daily commute to and from work, and a modest two-bedroom condo with no yard or greenspace for gardening. Moreover, we were done scraping by month after month feeling that we would never get 'ahead'. We wanted to create a life where our work felt fulfilling and inspiring and could grow and evolve as we did. We wanted to put energy into a business of our own that would create location freedom and improve our financial situation and overall lifestyle. We had a hope and dream and we were determined to make it happen.

Being driven, career-oriented, and action-taking individuals, we had a strong desire to accomplish something. We moved forward throwing every bit of energy we had at it. From June of 2016 to the summer of 2017 we spent every waking moment trying to build our business while continuing to work part-time day jobs, maintain the household, and raise our three-year-old son. The more time we invested into growing our business, the smaller and smaller the window of time for 'us' became. The boundaries we placed on our time were loose, to say the least. For most of that first year, we were so focused on getting our business off the ground that we lost connection to one another. We had lost sight of the importance of downtime and play.

Our dedication and focus proved to be great entrepreneurial traits, but they also led to some poor habits and routines. Working early mornings and late nights was not a recipe for success. Living in such a small condo meant that the bedroom doubled as our home office. This made 'shutting off' and 'shutting down' very challenging. In the effort to see our vision become reality, I got up at 5:30 most mornings and hopped onto the computer before my brain even had time to wake up. Many evenings, after our son was in bed, I spent long hours on my phone taking client calls or on the computer sending emails and writing marketing posts. Over time it began to take its toll.

A year into our business launch my body decided it had enough of the go, go, go. I was diagnosed with anemia. I was not doing a very good job of creating a work-life balance and my body was rebelling. My body has always had a way of 'messaging' me when something I was doing was not serving me; I just had to be sure to listen. In this particular situation, extreme fatigue was the message; not something I could easily ignore. I had run myself so ragged chasing after my dreams that my body forced me to stop and assess my health.

I recall crashing hard on the couch several afternoons a week while my son sat next to me watching 'Thomas the Tank Engine' DVD's. I needed time to recharge my batteries. I knew something wasn't right and I wasn't proud of the bad habits I had created. Lack of sleep, overwork, and lack of care for my physical needs had taken their toll. My wife and I had also been missing 'our time'– simply enjoying each other's company and connecting without the distraction of our business.

The good news is that with every breakdown comes a break-through. Mine was that the boundaries between my work, personal care, and family life were out of alignment. Shortly after learning about the anemia and getting on an iron supplement, I started to feel more like my high-energy self again. I knew that what we needed was to create better boundaries around our work hours and the time we spent on our devices. We needed to stop pushing and overworking ourselves. We needed to work smarter, not harder.

We created a better schedule that allowed us to get our work done without the burn-out. We worked six days a week with a more manageable schedule and always left Sundays for family time. We shut down each night by 8:30 pm to leave us more time for each other. These and other simple changes led to feeling more connected to each other, our work, and our long-term vision. Work was no longer allowed to compromise sleep. We made connecting a priority and it served us well. The best path to your goals is the one with a clear vision and well-established boundaries and ultimately it paid off in our business success, too.

DON'T BE A TECH SLAVE

Cell phones, tablets, mobile devices – call them what you will, they have become 'things' that most people cannot imagine living without. As a society we don't go very far without consulting them, using them, or playing on them. Remember that day when your phone went missing? That sinking feeling, like you'd lost everything? That frantic but unsuccessful search for it in your hand bag, back pack, under the couch, and all the usual 'drop spots'? Talk about an anxiety attack and high blood pressure! If you own a mobile device (as around five billion people do), you know all too well what I'm talking about.

We have become slaves to our devices. Without them we are literally lost. In a matter of minutes we can go from 'calm cool and collected' to highly agitated, full-on panic mode. Our phones alert us to our next event, our wake-up time, our lunch break, our kid's extracurriculars, our daily steps, and our messages, texts, and emails. Heck, thanks to Siri, they even talk back! Cell phones can now do just about anything you can think of. If we continue to spend time sitting at our desks and depending on our phones, there will soon be a built-in potty reminder. Laugh it up – but it's totally possible.

Numerous articles are being written by those taking a closer look at mental health and the effects our technologically-based world is having on us. We're seeing higher rates of depression, loneliness, sadness, and certain diseases among seniors. We're seeing higher rates of anxiety, weaker immune systems, and decreases in psychological and physical health. Across all age groups, people are struggling to manage their physical responses to stress and stressful events.

Spending endless amounts of time with our eyes pasted to a screen, our heads pigeoned forward (causing neck and back pain), and our butts warming an office chair is wreaking havoc on our bodies and minds. The medical community has come up with an informal term for this metabolic syndrome and the ill effects of an overly-sedentary lifestyle: 'sitting disease'.

According to several studies, the average person in the United States sits for 6.5 hours a day. For people aged 12 to 18 that number increases to eight or more hours a day. This includes time on a mobile device, computer, TV, commuting to and from work, sitting in class, or studying after class.

Face-to-face connection, even for as brief a time as a family meal once a day, has been proven to reduce the risk of teenage smoking, drinking, crime, depression, and other substance abuse. Of course, it also reduces the physical ailments that arise from always 'being on'. Rising physical inactivity in every demographic is leading to a host of illnesses and diseases. Sleep problems like insomnia and sleep apnea are more common. We're seeing more chronic aches, pains, hormone imbalances, and impaired focus, creativity, and productivity than ever.

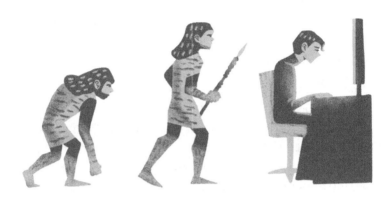

Eye strain and breakdowns in brain patterns and brain development are two other problems associated with excessive technology use. The choice to unplug is yours to make, and I hope you choose wisely.

Technology is both our salvation and our sentence: use it wisely.

I remember many in-depth conversations with my parents as a kid. They were filled with emotion and that emotional connection gave me so much feedback about the world around me that I would never have received through virtual messaging. We need this type of feedback in order to grow, respond, and take action in the world.

In-person interactions give us something virtual communication never can: the ability to read body language, receive communication stimuli, observe facial expressions and hand gestures, and recognize changes in voice tone. By connecting and communicating with others in real time, be it with your co-workers or your loved ones, your conversations are likely to be more thorough, positive, and productive. This type of connection also lends itself to more successful relationships.

How many hours a day do you find yourself mindlessly scrolling Facebook, Instagram, playing Candy Crush, or watching cat videos? Is it time to reevaluate how you spend your time? Might it be time to unplug? Has this behaviour become the acceptable way to 'zone out', 'chill', or 'reward yourself' after a long day, one that likely included many hours sitting in front of a computer? Are you ready to take a tech break?

Don't get me wrong – I'm all about enjoying *downtime*. I have a Netflix account, a Disney+ subscription, and I watch TV a few nights a week. But, from a health standpoint, I recognize when these behaviours are done in excess, they begin to intrude upon time to imagine, be creative, move our bodies, get out in nature, or connect with neighbours, family, and friends.

On top of its physical and emotional effects, consider the electromagnetic fields and radio frequencies that technology emanates. Government health and safety regulators have even deemed these rays as 'potentially carcinogenic to humans'. Total avoidance would be our best course of action but we all know this is not a realistic option. What is realistic is distancing ourselves, cutting back, and taking frequent breaks during the day to avoid too much tech time. Replace the time you spend connected to your phone, device, or TV screen with time spent really connecting with real people.

The message here is, don't be a tech slave. Place boundaries on your phone, gaming, or Netflix account. Choose ways to spend your time that light you up, connect you to others in real time, and improve your quality of life. We did not evolve through history with phones in our hands and buds stuck in our ears. This new way of life is impacting the way we function in the world, our own health, and that of our children. Unplug and get outside; these two simple tasks will improve your health immensely.

THEN AND NOW

When I was a kid, my friends and I spent our spare time climbing trees, biking, doing chores in and around the home, connecting with loved ones, friends, using our imagination, playing board games, creating art, and exploring the world around us. There were far more opportunities to just enjoy a little downtime without being overscheduled or glued to a screen.

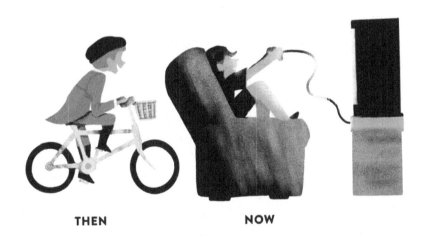

THEN   **NOW**

Fast forward to the present day. Many families live quite differently. Adults' and children's schedules are jam-packed with extracurricular activities. People are spending long hours at the office and then coming home to veg out on the couch because they're exhausted after a long day. What children and adults do for downtime often involves computers, video gaming, or watching TV. These habits and lifestyle choices leave very little space or opportunity to simply be: to dream, create, and move our bodies; to make believe, be silly, and let our minds wander off.

Far more than ever before, adults and children are suffering from things like depression, social anxiety, and fear of crowds and social interactions. They find it easier to hide behind a screen than to have a real-time conversation. Human connection is super important, yet technology is literally creating walls between us.

Did you know that our best ideas and most inspiring moments occur during times of play? Times when we are overcome with joy and pleasure? Moments when we are lost in thought, sports, movement, or a creative project. It's not when we are engaged with a computer, video game, or TV. You know those days (I hope you've had a few), when you lose track of time and your most inspirational and innovative ideas flood in. It's when we are so engaged and connected to who we are and the joy that life brings us, that we feel and live our happiest moments.

Seeds of creativity flourish when you set your mind free to dream, to wander, to simply be.

In order to create more connection to others, you first must carve out downtime to connect with yourself. The easiest way to do this is by sitting with your own thoughts and feelings without the need to be constantly 'consuming,' whether through social media, a Netflix series, or gaming. These past times are fun, but they also distract you from yourself. Connecting with yourself and others means putting down phones, powering off ipads, video games, and computers so that you can be fully present.

Another great way to feel a greater sense of connection to yourself is by connecting to your soul or spirit through quiet reflection, meditation or journaling, for example. (For a more in-depth discussion of connecting to the Self, see Chapter 6, Mindfulness.)

Connecting with others is about practicing active listening and conversing. It's about communicating with intention, and finding enjoyment in the company of your own thoughts and feelings, and those of other people. Given that one basic human need is for connection, it's paramount for our health and well-being to seek out opportunities that create downtime to power-off, play, and connect.

VIRTUAL CONNECTIONS

Do you remember what it was like, not so long ago, receiving a letter in the mail? Maybe you even had a pen pal as a kid? Historically, a good ol' pen and paper has been one of the most well-used forms of communication ever. The ability to put words on a page allowed for an entirely different form of communication and connection. As a kid, finding something addressed to me in the mailbox sent me over the moon. It still does to this day.

Living as we did in a rural community, our mailbox had a metal flag and stood on a pole at the end of the driveway. The mail person would drive up, drop the letters into the mailbox, and put up the flag, so we knew something had arrived. It feels like ages ago that snail mail was the norm. Written communication took weeks to arrive at its destination. Back then it was all we knew. Waiting for a letter or a parcel to arrive had its upside, though. It instilled patience and good communication – very different from our modern world.

Now we live at such a rapid pace we've grown accustomed to responses to text messages, emails, or phone calls arriving within minutes or even seconds of sending them. When we don't hear back from someone right away, we jump to conclusions. Are they upset with me? Did I say something to offend them? Is something wrong? Why aren't they getting back to me? We want instant gratification. Anything less may leave us plagued with self-doubt and wild projections and misconceptions.

What happened to the days of personal conversation? The days we actually picked up the phone and called someone? That left far less room to misinterpret what someone meant by their words because we got 'real-time' feedback. Back in the day we could easily gather more information about what was being said than we can now, due to tone of voice, emotion, and the silence between the words. When we called someone we could hear their voice, hear them laugh, cry, or share any other emotional charge that the conversation may have evoked.

Texting and emailing leaves little room for emotional connection. Sure emojis and gifs are fun, but we lose much of the personal part of communicating and connecting. Emails and texts are so often misinterpreted by the receiver; the emotion behind such messages is never genuinely felt. Having a real-time conversation with someone or, better yet, meeting them in the flesh builds a bond, a sense of community, and connectedness like no other.+

Listening is an act of appreciation. Appreciation builds strong communities, relationships, and connections.

As much as I love my iPhone, there are days when I would prefer to toss it out the window of a moving vehicle and never look back. I am on the fence as to whether or not I fully enjoy this age of social media, algorithms, Google, and emojis, or if my heart remains in the world of the rotary dial phone and converter box. In case you are reading this and were born after the 1980's, take a quick moment and look these things up! You will very quickly learn that the advances we've seen in such a short time are outstanding. Our digital media-based society and technological advances are happening at an astounding speed, and, like every-thing else in life, they carry both pros and cons.

On the plus side, they connect us like never before to new and old friends, family near and wide, and help keep us up-to-date on the goings-on around us. They provide opportunities to stay connected. They create location freedom in our jobs. Platforms like Skype, Zoom, and FaceTime help bring people together when it would otherwise be impossible. Major advances in the medical system are helping people recover from injury and illness better and faster.

Who doesn't love being able to use a single, hand-held device to take pictures at any place and time, shoot a video, check an email, get the weather forecast, Google something or someone, or play Scrabble with friends? It's brilliant in so many ways and it's forever improving. But online space also has a dark side. Things like cyber-bullying, information overload, fake news, and never-ending ads all have an impact on our mental health. FOMO (fear of missing out) is a real thing and affects many people.

Not only do our devices induce emotional turmoil, they cause physical ailments like finger, wrist, neck, and back pain, and over the long run, they promote a more sedentary lifestyle in people who use them to excess. Those aches and pains you get in your hand when texting? That's your body telling you you've been on your phone too long or too often.

Almost everything and anything can be done with a push of a button, or better yet, a voice command. Cleaning our clothes, washing our dishes, turning on our TV, our cars, and any other previously laborious jobs can now be done with minimal or no effort on our part. The advances that make daily life so much easier also equate to less physical exertion and more disease and illness. Not a great combo for the upcoming generations who are struggling to stay active, fit, and to manage things like stress, health ailments, depression, and anxiety.

Humans have the ability to be more connected (virtually) than ever before. Yet, at the same time, we're starved for human contact. We need and thrive on real-time, face-to-face human interactions. Research shows that human contact, like connection, is part of our hierarchy of needs. It's right up there with healthy eating and proper exercise. It supports the living of a long and happy life. Something as simple as a hug releases the hormone oxytocin, which in turn reduces stress, blood pressure, and anxiety.

People who choose to isolate themselves are far more at risk of depression, anxiety, a weakened immune system, obesity, cognitive decline, Alzheimer's disease, and even death. We need human contact to survive. Hiding behind a screen and avoiding social situations reduces your opportunities for human connection and ultimately your health.

Life is like a train travelling toward its destination. Be sure to get off at each stop or you will miss the journey.

THE BRIGHT SIDE OF TECH

With all the negative health effects the world is experiencing from advances in technology, there is still a bright side. COVID-19 has given rise to a global pandemic. In a matter of months the world has changed, perhaps forever, and in ways that nobody could have ever anticipated.

Living during a time like this has created a need for some very strict protocols and safety measures that affect not only our bodies, but our minds. Every single corner of the world has been sent into varying degrees of isolation.

What worries me most is how all of this is going to affect the psyche and long-term interaction between us, those around us, and the world at large. At the peak of the emergency, millions of people were required to stay home, unless leaving the house was absolutely necessary. Companies and local businesses moved employees from office buildings to their kitchen tables so work could 'continue as usual'. Only those considered 'essential workers' were allowed to move about the community, under strict guidelines and safety measures.

Parents have suddenly become employees, full-time caregivers, homeschooling teachers, and homemakers. Expectations for managing a wide range of responsibilities are rising and external support is falling. Stress levels have gone way up. Very few people leave home without a mask and hand sanitizer. We have seen an increase in depression, anxiety, anger, social isolation, and loneliness, all of which can worsen symptoms for those dealing with mental illness. It's just the way of the world in the 21st century.

With it all, our need for human connection is at an all-time high, and has prompted us to other measures that are both creative and drastic. Family trips across the country have been replaced with weekly FaceTime dates. Phone calls to family and friends that happened once in a while have become high priority. Work meetings, in-person events, and work once done 'in-person' have moved online. Some jobs have been created and others eliminated. Without technological advances, none of these connection points and changes would have been possible.

With all the uncertainty, it has become a very important time to reflect and connect. We have been forced to reflect on our lives, needs, health, financial situations, priorities, and long-term goals. Many of us have been stopped dead in our tracks as our lives have radically changed. On the flip side, many of us have had more quality time to spend with family members enjoying art, crafts, music, board games, time in nature, laughing, cooking, camping, and simply being together.

Despite the anxiety and challenges, I believe that living through a global pandemic has brought many of us closer together than anything else ever could. I believe it has taught us that nothing in life should be taken for granted: our food security, our health, our freedom of action, and everything we do to meet our need for physical, human connection.

Social distancing might stop people from gathering in large groups, but only for a time. Human connection is a need. It's thanks to major advances in technology that family and friends far and wide have had the opportunity to remain 'in touch' and connected as we all navigate this brand new world.

BLUE ZONES

Several years ago I stumbled upon an article about 'blue zone communities'. I was immediately intrigued, so I dug deeper. As it turns out, there are places in the world where people are living healthy lives, without reliance on medication, well into their well into their 90's and 100's. These places include the Italian island of Sardinia, Okinawa (Japan), Loma Linda (California), Costa Rica's remote Nicoya Peninsula, and Ikaria, an isolated Greek island.

I dug deeper still and learned that these people were not living longer because of some kind of secret lifestyle. It's actually because of something so simple that most people pay little atten-tion to. Their lifestyle emphasizes not only healthy eating, daily exercise, and minimal stress, but family connection, purposeful work, religion, and surrounding oneself with others who are of like mind. Community connection both improves our health and propels our lives.

It's possible for every one of us to find or create a community where human interaction, connection, trust, and love are at the forefront. Here are some simple ways to do that. Introduce your-self to your neighbours – the people on your street, your block, or condo building. Attend events in your community where you will see others, get to know them, and build a sense of connection and safety.

In 2018, our family moved into a townhome complex dating from the 1970's. Back then, homes were built to focus on community. Each of the 30 front doors faces into a beautiful common space with a grassy courtyard, trees, flowers, and a water fountain in the center. We quickly picked up the vibe that everyone knows everyone, something that felt important to us and our young family.

Although we all live our separate lives and go about our business day-to-day, if anyone needs anything (eggs, sugar, butter, someone to watch our kid while we make dinner, etc.), we have each other to rely on. This has created a true sense of community, safety, and security. Not only do I know 80% of my neighbours by name, but I know they are willing to look out for my home and my son at any given time. It's community at its best and we feel blessed to be experiencing it.

I believe that's what developing and living in a blue zone community is all about. You too can create this sense of connection and care in your neighbourhood but you must be willing to open up to the possibility – to say 'hi' to others, to introduce yourself, and to generate the connections you want and need.

Face to face interactions ignite the senses, creating opportunities for connection and love.

CONNECTION THROUGH MOVEMENT

When he was in Grade 1, my son brought home a drawing with a question at the top that read, 'What is your favourite thing?' A small amount of sadness filled my heart when I realized that what he had drawn was his 'game phone'. The sadness was because I would never have chosen this as my favourite thing when I was his age. It wasn't that I judged his decision; it just never crossed my mind that he would choose this above all else. Sheesh, he only got to enjoy the dang thing for 90 minutes a week. Had it really left that much of an impression on him? Was it really the Holy Grail of his world and the thing that brought him the most enjoyment? Where had we gone wrong? I know, I know, he was only six, but still! My wife and I had done a lot of groundwork work to ensure we had a solid family bond. There must be something else he loved?!

I share this story because truth be told, our kids are not the only ones who cherish, fixate on, and love their devices. My son gets tech time four days a week. Those are the times my wife and I allow him to enjoy one of his most desired pleasures. Given he lacks any kind of self-regulation, at least at this point, and his mood is affected by his time spent playing games, he still needs monitoring. Not only is it not the best use of his time but it also takes away from time to explore, imagine, and play with others.

The same is true for adults. Putting down your phone and walking away from your game of Candy Crush or Fortnite can be a challenge. How about those endless hours spent scrolling Facebook or Instagram? What can feel like minutes easily turns into hours. While numbing your brain and your body, you are losing valuable time to connect with the world around you. Am I saying you should never enjoy these things if they bring you pleasure? No. But I am saying that the choices you make around how to spend your time either improve your life or they don't.

According to research, those who sit behind desks or spend their spare time on their devices should aim to move their bodies at least every 30-60 minutes. Are you moving your body every 30-60 minutes that you sit at work or home?

Call me crazy, but I have dumbbells in my home office and a mini trampoline in the next room. I do my best to move my body at least every hour I'm in front of the computer. It resets my posture, gets blood flowing, and makes me more productive. It also gives me the chance to check in with my wife and son, step outside for natural sunlight, go to the bathroom or grab some more water.

I have the same routine with my son and his game time. He knows when I walk in the room to check on him that I'm going to ask him to get up and run around, go up and down the stairs, or do a few jumping jacks. That's the precedent that's been set. Our kids can get sore necks and backs too and we have to be the example. Placing some parameters around how often and how long you and your family spend on your devices will change your day and your mood.

If you find yourself strapped to your desk with no other options in sight I encourage you to consider a standing or walking desk. Many great options exist that help our bodies move more often, we just have to find which set-up is right for us and our workplace. If you work in a building with a set of stairs, use them. If there is green space or a walking path close by, take your lunch break on the road. Take a two-minute stretch, strength, or cardio break every hour. Enjoy meetings with colleagues or phone calls while on the move. Who said sitting in a boardroom for an hour was the most productive way to inspire your team and improve morale? There are endless ways to move more and sit less. So get creative and make it happen.

UNITE WITH MOTHER EARTH

Making human connections is important but we can take this one step further and look at the importance of regaining our connection to nature. When we do, we develop an even stronger connection to ourselves. With all the pressure and stress many of us carry in our lives it's easy to become separated or forget the importance of being in nature. It's easy to shift focus and make work our priority. And sadly, for most, work means sitting at a computer monitor (or two), in an office with artificial light, and closed windows. Because this environment lacks fresh air, natural light, and vegetation, people are developing some pretty interesting phobias and health challenges.

As a kid, I spent most of my waking hours outside riding my bike, hiking, playing in the dirt, jumping in puddles, swimming in the lake, or in winter, sledding and building a snowman. Most kids of my generation will have shared the same experiences. Playing outdoors was simply what we did. Research shows that most people do not spend more than 30 minutes outside each day. In some cases, it's their work that keeps them in; in other cases, they no longer want to be out. They are unsure of how to navigate the elements and prefer not to.

Case in point: a kid on my son's soccer team last summer was petrified of the wind. As I stood on the sidelines watching the game I observed his mother frantically trying to calm him down and shield him from the wind. He was having a full-on panic attack. I had never really given phobias and fears around nature much thought until that moment. Sure, I've got my fears of things like snakes or big hairy spiders, but I still find them fascinating and enjoy observing them (from a distance).

I believe that when we spend so many hours indoors that we lose our connection to the natural world, the very cloth from which we are made. There are some really good practices for rebuilding and maintaining a connection to the soil, water, wind, and woods. *Earthing** (or 'grounding') is one of my favourites. The earth holds a magnetic charge that helps to ground us. Because we wear shoes most of the time, we block that energy from penetrating our bodies.

Therefore, earthing is simply being outside with your shoes and socks off. You can absorb the earth's grounding energy in as little as 20 minutes. (Twenty minutes twice a day is recommended, but any amount is better than none at all.) Start with five minutes a day, and work up. By making this a daily practice, you can reap the earth's bounty at no cost whatsoever. Like I've said before, doing something consistently is better than putting a timestamp on something but never actually doing it.

Numerous studies confirm the healing benefits of earthing. It has been found to improve sleep and immunity, and to decrease stress, cortisol levels, and pain. It has also been found to neutralize free radical damage to our cells from things like trauma and environmental toxins. Free radicals wreak havoc in our bodies, and lead to a host of health concerns and autoimmune conditions.

So head on out right now. Walk through the grass in your yard or at the park. Head over to the beach and walk along the shore line or through the sand barefoot. See for yourself the energy and pleasure that come with connecting to the earth.

Dip your toes in the ocean. Wade along the sands. Stroll through the grass. Hug a tree.

Another fantastic way to connect more with nature is through *forest bathing**. I have been a hiking fan since I was a kid. I always found the forest such a magical and comforting place. I especially love the fall when the leaves change colours and the wind blows through the branches above, creating a soft clicking noise. It's soothing and peaceful. There is something mystical about being among the trees, the sounds of nature, the earth below my feet, the smells, and the colourful trees. It's serenity at its best.

Through my research I learned that the concept of forest bathing or *shinrin-yoku* originated centuries ago in Japan. The term *shinrin* means 'forest' and *yoku* means 'bath'. The concept is that we are able to take in the forest atmosphere through our senses. When we spend time in nature we are able to connect to the earth through the use of sight, smell, hearing, taste, and touch. This method of living has been thought of as a way to bridge the gap between us and nature.

I was well into my 30's before I was introduced to the concept of forest bathing. I had been enjoying the forest all my life but didn't realize I could take it to the next level and embrace it with a new-found consciousness. Numerous studies have been done proving the health benefits associated with being among the trees. The most notable benefits of forest bathing are how it eases stress and worry, and helps us relax and think with greater clarity. It also boosts mood and energy while creating a sense of vitality as it refreshes and rejuvenates us. In addition to the physical health benefits, time in the forest creates a sense of comfort.

The next time you head out for a hike or adventure in the woods, take some time to connect. Observe how you feel in your body and mind. It's the cheapest and one of the most effective ways to reduce anxiety and create a sense of calm. Take a few deep breaths into your belly, smell the air, listen to the sounds, hug a tree, eat some fresh berries (be sure they're not poisonous), and put yourself in touch with nature. Whether you choose to take a forest bath for exercise, mental health, or to improve your connection to nature, the benefits are endless and immediate.

IN CONCLUSION

There are three main elements of connection: connection to yourself, connection to others, and connection to the world around you. Connecting to yourself means tuning into your inner voice, noticing what your body needs, and accepting your thoughts and emotions. Connecting to others is about building relationships, being a good listener, and finding enjoyment in sharing time together, be it in-person or through virtual channels. Connection to the world around you means exploring and appreciating the beauty of nature and all that it brings to your life. When each of these aspects of connection are felt and lived, they can improve your emotional, physical, and mental health, and do the same for those around you.

THE SUCCESS OF HUMAN CONNECTION

Tina's Story

Tina is a mom to two teenagers. She and her family spent nearly all of their free time glued to their devices. Things had not always been this way, but as her kids got older it slowly became the norm. Only rarely did they just hang out together, enjoying each other's company, as they once had. Each seemed to have become very caught up in their own lives and intimate family time fell way down their list of priorities.

In Tina's home after 4 pm, everyone was glued to a device, doing their 'own thing'. Although Tina had fallen as deeply into this pattern as her husband and kids, what she really wanted was to change it. She wanted to go back to the times when her family connected over a meal, enjoyed some simple conversation, or went for a walk together.

On one of our coaching calls Tina mentioned that it felt as if her family, specifically her teenagers, were set in their ways. She was unsure how to break these routines without major protest. Since her hubby enjoyed his zone-out evening screen time just as much as the kids, it was even harder to implement changes, despite her best intentions.

After getting a better understanding of what Tina really wanted more of in her life, we discussed some options to help re-establish the situation at home and her family's connection to one another. We talked about how hard change can be and that things might not go seamlessly, but that she shouldn't give up on it. We also came up with a few ways to get the 'buy-in' she needed from her family. I suggested she start by being honest and telling them why setting aside quality time for one another mattered so much to her.

We discussed a variety of possibilities: planning a trial period and re-assessing; making the change to evening patterns a group effort; and setting clear boundaries to which everyone could contribute and commit. It really came down to having some good communication and honesty.

As you know, human beings are very quick to develop routines and habits. Breaking them feels difficult but it doesn't have to be. I warned Tina that the kids might show resistance. If she was to succeed, she had to communicate what she needed and wanted while still giving her family the space to contribute to the plan. It was a great tool to evoke empathy, develop good communication, and strengthen their family bond.

The night after our coaching call was game-changing. For the first time in a long time Tina spoke to her family about her desires for connection, about what it would mean to her, and asked for their opinions. Things were going so well that she asked her family if they could commit to a no-device rule between 5 and 7 pm five days a week. She told them how much she missed hearing how their days had gone or sharing with them about her day. She missed laughing and reminiscing about the past. She also shared how much she enjoyed her downtime on her device, but recognized how important it was to carve out a few hours each day to spend together.

It took courage and willpower for Tina to ask for what she needed and follow through on the plan. Initially, there was some resistance. But she reminded herself that it was going to take time for everyone to see and feel the benefit of their new evening routines.

In the weeks to follow, they all came to the conclusion that hanging out as a family for two hours each evening was totally doable, and in fact, enjoyable (even if it was not always their first choice). Clear parameters and expectations were a big part of the family's success. Each night at 5 pm all of their phones had to go into a basket on the counter and stay there, untouched until 7 pm. And they did it!

It was a big, yet simple step for everyone. They created two hours dedicated to connection: prepping dinner together, conversation, a family walk, a card game, or simply being together without distraction. It was the precious family time that had been missing for each of them and they appreciated getting it back.

Tina put in place a simple plan that made connecting with family a top priority. This one small shift will continue to have a profound impact on her relationship with her kids and her husband. She is proud of her efforts and those of her family, and so am I!

4
—

NUTRITION

*T*here's a lot of noise out there when it comes to eating and nutrition. There are many companies vying to convince you that following their *diet** plan is the best way to lose weight. Maybe they have supplements and a prepackaged weight-management system that make health 'as quick and easy as 1-2-3.' The truth is, when it comes to health, quick fixes are a trap. The best way to improve your lifestyle, lose weight, gain muscle, or achieve any other health-related goal is to make sustainable eating choices each and every day.

More about sustainable eating later. To get started, let's talk about why people eat in the first place. Most times you likely eat because your body tells you that you're hungry, and stop when it tells you that you're full. Kids are really good at listening to those cues. They eat more when they're hungry, then stop when they are full, instead of eating to the point of discomfort.

But people eat for other reasons, too. Let's take a closer look at why people eat when they are *not hungry*.

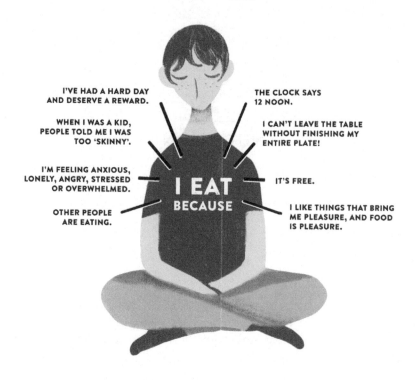

I'VE HAD A HARD DAY AND DESERVE A REWARD.

WHEN I WAS A KID, PEOPLE TOLD ME I WAS TOO 'SKINNY'.

I'M FEELING ANXIOUS, LONELY, ANGRY, STRESSED OR OVERWHELMED.

OTHER PEOPLE ARE EATING.

THE CLOCK SAYS 12 NOON.

I CAN'T LEAVE THE TABLE WITHOUT FINISHING MY ENTIRE PLATE!

IT'S FREE.

I LIKE THINGS THAT BRING ME PLEASURE, AND FOOD IS PLEASURE.

I EAT BECAUSE

EATING FOR THE RIGHT REASONS

The goal for all of us (and not just those who want to shed some weight) is to listen to our bodies: eat when we are hungry and stop when we are full. For some people this is much easier said than done. The stomach shrinks or expands based on the quantity of food ingested on a regular basis. A typical human stomach is the size of your fist. That's not very big. That's why understanding whether your body needs food or fluids is helpful in maintaining a healthy body weight.

Did you know that your body's cue for hunger feels the same as its cue for thirst?

I know, it's a bit unfair, but it's the truth. That's one good reason to drink a glass of water at the onset of hunger. It helps to hydrate you, and it will curb that hunger pang in the event you're just thirsty. Drinking water between meals is another good habit to adopt. It keeps you hydrated while suppressing your sensation for hunger, so you overeat less often. Keeping a routine around the times of day you eat will also help your body get into a rhythm about when to expect food and drink and when not.

Nourishing your body means living without judgment, deprivation, or restriction.

Eating more mindfully is the first step to a better understanding of your body. So drink that full glass of water or herbal tea and wait five minutes. If you still feel hungry, then opt for a snack or meal.

Another way to avoid erratic hunger pangs is to limit the amount of time between your meals. Three to five hours may be an ideal time frame, depending on what you eat. Anything longer will put your body into 'starvation mode': your blood sugar goes out of whack, your mood changes, your energy drops, and you may even become 'hangry'. Remember the last time you were so hungry you were angry?! I know you feel me. When too many hours go by without food, you are more prone to gobble up anything within reach, as if you're a caveman who doesn't know when to expect the next meal. It's a survival tactic that we've long outgrown, but remains built-in, like wisdom teeth.

OK. It's confession time. I did not realize how much my choices and motivation around preparing, cooking, and eating healthy meals would be influenced by having a child in the house. I have enjoyed eating home-cooked and healthy meals for many years. But setting a good example, even when I'm tired and don't feel like cooking, matters more now that a little person is looking to me (and my wife) for guidance about what's right and wrong. Food habits are a huge part of that. One day he brought home a school art project in which he had drawn his favourite meal. He drew a salad with tomatoes and cucumbers, yam fries, ketchup, and a glass of water. So I'm pretty sure the messages he's been receiving since he was a babe are sinking in. Go veggies!

Like most parents, I want my son to grow up with a sense of what a well-balanced meal looks like. For sure we have pancakes for dinner occasionally; it's just not the norm. The other factor that influences my motivation is my wife. She grew up in a home with a well-balanced meal (and no dessert) on the table each night. Her idea of dinner includes a protein, a carb, and some vegetables. Most nights I'm game for a good solid meal, but at least once a week a few slices of toast with peanut butter and banana or a bowl of cereal can be totally satisfying. That was a snack I enjoyed with my mom when I was a kid. Way less mess in the kitchen and my need for comfort food is totally met.

It's not that I don't love making dinner or feeling fueled and nourished. It's just that, because I have others who are deferring to me and counting on me, I'm more inclined to provide hot, home-cooked dinners more often. So even though I totally enjoy a carb-rich dinner with minimal cooking once in a while, I feel more nourished and energized because of my healthier habits.

The point here is that old patterns stick around even when we think we've moved beyond them. That slice of toast or bowl of cereal that I ate as a child has remained my 'go-to' evening snack. It brings me back to my childhood; it's my comfort food. There's nothing wrong with my choices, nor do I feel the need to change them. It really comes down to listening to my body, eating when I'm hungry, and making the best choices I can, most of the time. I encourage you to do much the same.

Back in Chapter 1, I told you about the high sugar diet that I came to crave in my late teens and early 20's. Over the past decade I have developed a better relationship with food, how I treat my body, and the cues it provides me. I started to eat for the 'right' reasons. That's the insight that I hope you take from this chapter. Eating for the right reasons means you will be better able to maintain your weight, lose weight, and support your body's needs for nourishment. 'Eating for life' (instead of 'living to eat') is a great philosophy to live by.

DISORDERED EATING

At the age of 19, a time in my life when so much seemed beyond my control or understanding, there were two things that I felt I could control: what I ate and how much I exercised. In my attempts to control them I developed some bad habits around food. For just shy of two years (two of the most difficult in my life), I suffered from anorexia nervosa. At the time, I did not fully comprehend what was happening to me. Several years later I realized that the eating disorder was my desperate attempt to gain some control of my life as I navigated my sexual orientation. My confusion led me down a slippery slope cluttered with many self-sabotaging decisions.

I believe that my poor relationship with food was triggered by a fear of who I was. What I longed for was self-acceptance of my body and of my lifestyle. What I needed was to change my relationship with myself so that I could improve my relationship with food. I knew that if I could change one, I would be able to change the other.

I will never forget those long and depressing days when baby carrots, rice cakes, dry bagels, and jars of baby fruit purée were all I ate. I recall feeling tired, weak, constipated, sad, and scared. I wanted to stay thin. I wanted to be noticed. I had this idea that if I was thin, people would like me more and I would attract more attention. I also thought it would lead to more happiness and acceptance from those around me. Those were the stories I told myself to justify my actions.

My monthly cycle stopped completely for one and a half years. I had literally run myself so deeply into the ground that my body's hormones could not function, a set of circumstances that continues to haunt me over 20 years later. When trapped in a cycle of negativity and self-destruction, there are certain things you can't see or if you can, that you simply are unwilling to look at.

If you've been down this road, you know what I'm talking about. It's like a wave that crashes down and keeps pulling you back under as you desperately try to climb out onto the shore. Those were some dark, lonely times – times that I would never wish on anyone nor ever want to experience again.

Yet, it was during those bleak days that I realized what emotional eating really is. Whenever I 'thought' I ate too much, I was filled with guilt, shame, and fear. Whenever I ate too little (which was most days), I felt depleted and craved more, yet I made sure to keep food at a distance. It wasn't easy and it wasn't fun but that was how I coped. Eating became an ongoing emotional battle.

Disordered eating can take many forms. Whether you struggle with bulimia, binge eating, anorexia, or another form of disordered eating, please know that support exists. Although the word 'eating' is in the name, these disorders are about so much more than food. They're mental health conditions that in most cases require medical intervention and psychological support. I share my story openly and honestly to encourage anyone who might be suffering to know you don't have to fight your battle alone. You can get through this. It will take willingness and time. I know. Those default patterns still creep back into my life from time-to-time even 20 years later.

Whatever food challenges you face, I wish you utmost love and strength. We will examine *body image** and my story in more detail in Chapter 6, Self-Love.

During my time of breakdown, I learned that I was going about finding acceptance and love in the wrong way. I was in a down-ward spiral that I could not climb out of. It was dark and it was depressing. I didn't like who I was but I didn't know how to self-correct. At least, not yet. I was insecure with my body and uncomfortable with my choices. It was in my early 20's that I finally came to a place of surrender. I slowly began my journey of accepting the person I really was. As I came to terms with who I was, I came to terms with who I wanted to be. I wanted to be strong, not weak. I wanted to be healthy, not skinny. This process helped me understand that food was not the enemy.

I started working with a counsellor, studying nutrition, and surrounding myself with people who accepted me just as I was. I learned that although our genetics can influence our body type and predisposition to being overweight, we are not products of our circumstances.

We have the ability to alter our own level of health. *We* get to choose how *we* nourish and care for our bodies. *We* decide how active *we* are and what *we* feed our minds.

This understanding helped shift my thinking. I knew I had not been doing a good job of caring for my body or my mind up to that point. I chose to leave that path. I began to forge a new one that provided me with hope for a healthier future. I realized the importance of the relationship between me and my body, and was willing to work on it. Nourishing my body became a part of my lifestyle.

EATING IS EMOTIONAL

For the vast majority of people, eating is emotional. We are hardwired to have an emotional reaction to and from food. Growing, meal planning, buying, prepping, smelling, seeing, hearing, touching, and the actual act of eating food, all provoke an emotional response from us. These responses give us feedback, pleasure, and connect us to our bodies, the earth, and those around us.

Experts define *emotional eating** as 'the consumption of food without hunger'. Food has the ability to trigger happy, positive, and pleasurable experiences. Like when you sit down to a meal with your family at Thanksgiving and you are overcome with gratitude. Or when you make yourself a breakfast that is full of nourishment and you feel good about your body and your choices. Or when you grab an ice cream cone and walk the beach strip and are immediately reminded of a happy memory from your childhood. These are all great ways in which food triggers emotion and makes you feel happy.

On the flip side, sadly, many people carry negative emotions when it comes to food and eating. For example, guilt around the choice of food they are consuming. Shame around their body that leads to self-loathing. Embarrassment that accompanies overeating or undereating, especially if someone notices and speaks to it. Even fear, because they don't want to be 'one of those difficult people' when they mention they have a food intolerance, sensitivity, or allergy.

The very thought of preparing food for yourself or your family, and then eating it, either stimulates feelings of happiness and satisfaction, or makes you feel stressed and anxious. We each carry with us our own food stories. These stories could be from our childhood, or the first time we lived alone, or maybe weekly dinners with our grandparents. Just like music and smells, food evokes a host of emotions and memories. Our emotions are very closely linked to our food associations and our habits. And this is okay! It is not something we can change.

What we can do is try to understand our body's needs and our own personal needs, what actually triggers different emotions, and leads us to eat. Food can be a way to self-soothe, fill a void, create a feeling of 'fullness' or temporary wholeness, and distract us from what is really going on. A better understanding of why we do what we do enables us to unpack these emotions and find other ways to create a similar emotional response, without taking a single bite. Until we gain that understanding, it can be very difficult to acknowledge, detach, release judgment, and make different choices about food.

Many of the factors that lead a person to eat can be more about emotion than hunger. Here are the main ones:

- Turning to food during times of emotional need, and neglecting to reach out for social support.
- Turning to food to release stress or improve your mood, for lack of interest in engaging in activities that might offer the same benefit.
- Turning to food because what you take to be physical hunger is actually an emotional response to hunger.
- Binge eating because of a vicious cycle of negative self-talk that leads to self-sabotage.
- Craving food due to hormonal changes, specifically cortisol, during times of stress.
- Eating mindlessly (without care or attention) due to anger, fear, or boredom.

In each of these situations, your body is flooded with emotions that, in the absence of alternatives, are soothed by food. Consciously or unconsciously, food becomes your habitual 'got-to'. You eat without hunger.

Here are five steps you can use to help you honour your emotions while choosing a new way to self-soothe.

Step 1

Learn and know your triggers. Do you mindlessly eat when you're stressed, overwhelmed, sad, lonely, happy, or 'deserve' a reward?

Step 2

Build a toolkit and use it. What tools do you have at your disposal to help simulate the feeling of 'wholeness' or satisfaction that food gives? Do you need connection with a loved one? Do you need a short walk and fresh air to blow off steam? Do you need to meditate or recite a positive affirmation to shift your focus from negative to positive?

Have a list of tools handy to support you in your moments of weakness or hire a coach or mentor to help you find what works for you.

Step 3

Practice releasing judgment. Accepting and letting go of any self-judging thoughts or feelings will help you avoid beating yourself up and feeling worse. Diving deep into a pit of despair, shame, or guilt will only perpetuate the cycle. Feel what you feel, and release judgment.

Step 4

Accept what is, congratulate yourself, and move on. It's hard to change old patterns and habits. They become ingrained in us and hold on even when we desperately want to be rid of them. That is why it's very important to honour your feelings, celebrate your wins, make conscious choices in a positive direction, and move forth without guilt or shame. Remember the last time you felt this way and how, instead of jumping to food, you shifted gears and made a different choice. Celebrate how well you took care of your body and/or mind that time.

Step 5

Rinse and repeat.

Personalized coaching is very helpful when dealing with nutrition and emotional eating. Your circumstances and needs around food are different from those of friends and family members, and cannot be addressed by or condensed into a single paragraph.

It's important to see your doctor if you feel that your eating patterns are beyond your control and my suggestions have not offered significant relief. Your doctor or therapist would be in a better position to know what is needed to navigate your habits beyond this book.

Ready to consciously choose self-love over self-sabotage? Find the link to my free *Body, Mind & Soul Snacking Survival* guide in the resources section. It will help you navigate some of the biggest emotional-eating triggers in a body-positive, self-loving, and conscious way. I encourage you to drop any guilt and shame you may carry around food and begin embracing it for the nourishment and joy it brings to your life.

What I eat fuels my body and my mind.

LET'S TALK ALCOHOL

I write about this subject with profound compassion and empathy. Alcohol has affected many of my extended family members and it was the primary cause of my biological father's passing. Copious amounts of alcohol, combined with years of smoking, permanently scarred his liver. He died of cirrhosis of the liver, among several other complications, at the age of 50.

Drinking alcohol as a way to unwind after a long day has become common practice for many people. I am not against enjoying a few drinks each week, but when alcohol becomes a daily occurrence, it's time to take a closer look at your choices and habits, and their long-term effects on your well-being.

I'm not here to tell you that you should or should not drink. However, what I am here to do is educate you on alcohol's impact on your body. In its most basic form, alcohol (ethanol or ethyl alcohol) is the ingredient found in beer, wine, and spirits that causes drunkenness, among other reactions. Ethyl alcohol is something your body recognizes as an invader and toxic substance and therefore its main goal is to get rid of it. Although alcohol contains a high caloric value (seven calories per gram), the body is able neither to reap any nutritional value from these calories nor store the energy for later use, unlike proteins (four calories per gram), fats (nine calories per gram), and carbohydrates (four calories per gram).

When alcohol enters your body, your stomach and liver immediately go to work to metabolize it. The liver, given its close proximity to the stomach, plays the biggest role because its job is to eliminate toxic substances, like ethanol, from your body. The liver is responsible for metabolizing 90% of the ethanol that you drink. That's a sizable workload for the liver, hence it's crucial to go easy on your body's biggest and most important defender against toxification.

Because of the body's inability to store ethanol, all other bodily processes must slow down until the ethanol has been moved along. That means that your body shifts from a state of concentration and focus into a state of relaxation and euphoria. Sure, it might be nice to feel your body become warm and relaxed but all its other systems are getting compromised as a result. Even your immune system and resting metabolism slow down. If weight loss, improved metabolic function, and overall well-being are your goal, alcohol is not your ally. In fact, it's a suppressant.

Take my client Josie, for example. When she and I first started coaching she disclosed that alcohol was ruling her life and had been for many years. It was affecting her motivation to move, her desire to make healthier food choices, her after-work habits, and the people with whom she spent time. She was running a successful business, raising three kids, and, since her husband worked out of town, spent many of her evenings alone, enjoying several glasses of wine while vegging out in front of the TV.

I made a few recommendations for support with her drinking (Alcoholics Anonymous and therapy), as this was not my scope of practice. However, she was certain that she had the ability to stop drinking at any time if she was in the right headspace, had the right support system, and wanted to stop badly enough. She had been down this road before and knew that the time had come to kick the habit. Josie wanted long-term change and she was determined to create new and healthier habits that did not revolve around evening bottles of wine.

Within the first month of coaching, and working together Josie lost ten pounds. The biggest contributor to her weight loss, at least initially, was that she replaced most of her evening wine with sparkling water. She got creative, adding things like lime or mint to her water to make it more like a cocktail. She committed to drinking only on weekends, and then only moderately. This was the shift she needed to start seeing progress in her body as well as her mind.

In the months to follow, not only did Josie's weight continue to drop, but she also began to experience greater focus, better sleep, and a stronger desire and motivation to exercise and cook healthy meals for herself and her family. She began meal planning and getting more organized, which made healthier habits easier to create. She replaced her evening Netflix habit with 30-minute workouts or walks with her dog. She enjoyed her hot tub as a reward after a long day instead of poor food choices, fatty snacks, and booze. She went to bed earlier and without the need for alcohol. This meant she woke up earlier feeling more energized. She started her day with a clear head and another walk with the dog, instead of hitting the snooze button until the very last second. This made for calmer mornings, with far less of the rush and anxiety that she had felt previously.

By tweaking a few small things, Josie's life had changed for the better. Alcohol and social drinking was still a part of her lifestyle and that was something she would have to address, on her terms. But they no longer dominated her life. I realize that there are many layers to drinking and alcoholism and no two situations are exactly alike. What I do hope you take from this, is that alcohol is a hindrance to your health and well-being, especially if you have weight loss goals. It affects your body and mind in ways you may not have even appreciated before. If you have reached a place where you want to change your habits and need support to do so, please seek it out. There is no shame, only love and encouragement here. Your liver will thank you!

PORTION IT

You've heard the stories of our ancestors scouring the land in search of food. They went days between meals and ate what they could find to survive. Those stories have never been our story. An abundance of food magically finds its way to the grocery store shelf. All we have to do is drive there and choose from an array of options that we then bring home and eat. No hunting, no major physical exertion, and no stress required, except maybe when we confront a long line-up or occasionally an 'out-of-stock' sign where our favourite flavour of yogurt generally sits.

The concept of eating proper portions for your body type and level of activity is simple and effective. It's not about cutting calories, omitting entire food groups, or depriving yourself of things you enjoy eating. It's more about eating the right amount of food for your body type and activity level. It's about ensuring you fill your plate, but not so full that you're busting at the seams. It's about understanding what your body needs and fueling it.

Even too much of a good thing can be a bad thing.

Regardless of whether you choose an overabundance of fast food or an overabundance of home-made quinoa salad, if your body is regularly fed more energy than it needs, it will store the excess. And you don't get to choose where that extra energy is stored. When I ask new clients about their eating habits, it's a loaded question. Some say, 'I eat really well,' yet they still struggle with weight loss. Some say, 'I'm following the Keto diet, but I've hit a plateau; it was working for a while and now it's not.' Others tell me straight up that their eating habits are the pits or that they overindulge regardless of food choices and they need help.

No matter what scenario you fall into, you can benefit from a clear yet simple understanding of portions and why they matter. When we eat the 'right foods' in the 'right amounts' for our bodies every day, we get the nutrients and energy we need to thrive.

Here's a tool that I learned from Precision Nutrition Inc. that you can integrate into your life seamlessly. It's a simple way to estimate how big a serving of each food group your body needs at meal-time. If you are eating to maintain a healthy lifestyle, then eat serving sizes as suggested here, aiming for three meals a day. If weight loss is your goal, then reduce the amount of each serving slightly. In addition to providing easily maintainable serving sizes, this tool helps ensure that your body gets the nutritional value it needs for optimal functioning. It takes into account each food group and the nutrients associated with it.

THE HAND METHOD

THIS IS A SIMPLE AND EFFECTIVE WAY TO MEASURE FOOD AND
NUTRIENTS BASED ON YOUR BODY SIZE. MOST PEOPLE'S HANDS
ARE PROPORTIONAL TO THEIR BODY MAKING THIS METHOD
DISCREET AND EASY TO USE. IT ALSO SAVES YOU FROM
COUNTING OR TRACKING CALORIES AND QUANTITIES.

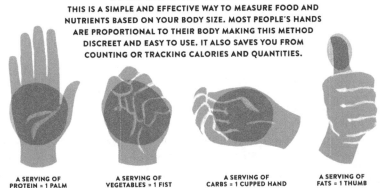

A SERVING OF PROTEIN = 1 PALM   A SERVING OF VEGETABLES = 1 FIST   A SERVING OF CARBS = 1 CUPPED HAND   A SERVING OF FATS = 1 THUMB

I find it helpful to think of the body like a car. If you drive your car a lot, you need more fuel to make it go. You need more rest, recovery, and maintenance. If you neglect your car, or forget to get an oil change or to do routine maintenance, it will break down. If you let your car sit for long periods of time, the parts become brittle, tires go flat, the fuel gums up, and rust sets in. The same is true of our bodies. We need fuel to go, but not too much, or the tank overflows. We need regular maintenance to keep us healthy and we need to move each day for optimal functioning. Give your car what it needs and it will hum along happily.

COUNT WHAT MATTERS

A lot of the counting done nowadays to assess health is a waste of time and effort. Whether it's calories, macros, micros, points, kilos, or steps, many common measures of health are unhelpful, at best. Sure, counting has its place. Elite athletes trying to meet their weight class, or someone who wants to improve lean muscle tissue for a competition, or someone with diabetes, who needs to keep their blood sugar low – all these people are well-served by counting.

For the common person, however, counting drives you crazy. Especially in relation to eating habits. Counting can and will make 'that number' an obsession; you get hyper-focused on it while neglecting what your body is actually telling you. It's tedious and time-consuming, and not an endeavour that anyone can sustain their whole life long.

The fact is, it took you years to get where you are. A 'quick fix' is no solution to a long-term problem; in fact, it only makes the problem worse. You lose 20 pounds, only to gain back 25. This is defeating and down-right frustrating. In addition, it has a massive impact on your metabolism, hormones, and immune system and increases your risk for cardiac distress.

Maybe you're a numbers person. I get that. Count away, but turn your attention to other 'measurables', like how many minutes you spent moving your body today. Count the amount of weight you lifted in a single squat. Count the number of servings of vegetables you consumed today, or how long you held a plank exercise. Count the amount of time you spent on self-care, meditation, and self-improvement, or the number of loops you had to punch in your belt over the past year because your pants have been falling down. These are the numbers worth tracking because they measure long-term improvements in your lifestyle, strength, and overall health.

Balancing your health can feel like a numbers game. Be sure you're focusing on the right ones.

FOOD VS. FOOD PRODUCTS

Have you ever looked for a label on an apple, a carrot, or a bunch of kale? You won't find one, unless you buy a bag of apples or carrots. Otherwise, food in your grocery store's produce department does not come labelled. It's a whole food packed with nutrients whose relevance and importance to nourishing our bodies requires no itemization. Although some people believe apples 'come from the store', we all know that fresh, nourishing foods are grown from the earth, just the way mother nature intended.

We don't question the high nutritional value of something that grows in the soil, on a tree, or that we purchase directly from the farm. It's a given. We just know it's the healthiest choice.

Around 1910 food was well on its way to industrialization and was being produced in factories far from consumers. Processed and pre-packaged foods became the new thing. Food as we once knew it was being altered from its natural state and going through a refining process. Things like high levels of salt, MSG, and preservatives, as well as sugars and corn syrup were added to prolong the shelf life of food. Then it was popped into a nice package with a fancy label. As time passed, packaging and marketing got more sophisticated and eye-catching, and people bought into this 'new way' of buying and eating food. Packaged foods claimed to make our lives 'easier', cleaner, and even healthier in some cases.

One of my 'favourite' labels was the one that made Santa Claus famous: 'Vigorously good - and keenly delicious. Thirst quenching and refreshing.' It was put on bottles of Coca-Cola, one of the most addictive sodas on the market. It gained popularity and claimed to be 'everybody's drink'. Then came labels with slogans like 'low fat', implying that eating a diet low in fat was healthy.

What those labels failed to explain was that when fat was removed, so was flavour. In order to recreate a product that actually tasted good and that people wanted to eat, something had to be added.

How about 'ready to eat' food labels? As if taking the time to make a home-cooked meal was the worst thing you could do for yourself and your family. These false ideas have led us down a path of unhealthy choices, and it's only gotten worse as the years go by.

It's not hard to see why so many people are confused about the food industry, what's 'good food', what's not, and how to manage food cravings and addictions. It was during my mid-20's that I finally woke up. I started to question things instead of accepting them as they were. I recall pondering why man-made *food products** are so popular if they all lead to illnesses like heart disease, stroke, diabetes, and cancer. These foods are as high in risk as they are low in nutrients, yet we buy them every week in our grocery stores.

Am I saying never have pre-packaged, processed food? No, not at all. I too buy boxed cereal, crackers, and granola bars, but they're not something I choose every day. What I am saying is that eating a ratio of 80% whole foods and 20% processed will help you maintain your health and longevity.

The earth's abundance is the catalyst to life and longevity.

I first ventured out to a local farm in my mid 20's, built a relationship with a wonderful family that grew and prepared the food, and started learning about food – real food. That was also when I gained a new appreciation for vegetables, herbs, and free-range and organic growing systems. My mind was blown. There were so many fresh foods I had never even heard of, let alone eaten, like arugula, collards, kale, Swiss chard, and yams! I felt like a child in an ice cream parlour. A whole new world of fresh-food choices, endless in number, opened up before me.

With that opening, came a greater understanding and appreciation for food quality and security, a new way of buying and eating, and of course, improved health. I took cooking classes, researched produce items I knew nothing about, and started eating to thrive.

No matter how you were raised or what your current food habits and choices are, there is always room for improvement. I believe many of the world's illnesses can be reversed, or at the very least better managed, if people simply move away from processed food products to a diet rich in whole foods.

Food products are defined as 'substances that can be used or prepared as food.' Let that thought sink in for a moment. Most food products simply act as fillers, void of any substantial nutritional value. Is that really what you want from the food that goes into your body? These options may make our lives easier, but at what cost to our bodies and to the world?

The next time you prepare your meal plan and head off to the grocery store (or better yet, the farmer's market), please consider the following:

- View the produce section as if it's your best friend. Load up your cart with fresh produce first.
- Read food labels. If a label has more than four or five ingredients, look around for an alternative. Many processed foods contain preservatives and chemicals to keep them shelf stable, not for the sake of nourishing a human body.
- Be mindful of food labels that list ingredients you cannot pronounce. It's not likely to be a super-awesome vitamin or mineral you've never heard of. Lots of preservatives that can make us sick are disguised with fancy names.
- Seek out whole grain breads and cereals that have a value of four grams of fibre or more. This indicates less processing and our bodies need fibre each day for proper bowel health.
- Shop in the bulk section to save money on things like nuts, seeds, dried fruits, beans, legumes, and flour.

Grocery shopping, once a chore for me, has turned into a fact-finding expedition. A better understanding of how you want to feel and how you're going to get there can shift not only your perspective on food, but your buying habits.

Finally, take note of how many food products you buy and start making the transition to more whole-food, nutrient-dense options, one week at a time. No need to overhaul your life all at once. Small steps create big gains. When you start eating real food, take note of how your body feels. How much energy you have, improved bowel function (so important), your digestion, your ability to regulate hunger and satiety, and your overall outlook on eating and food. I guarantee that you will experience change as you shift from processed options to whole foods.

MINDFUL EATING

One of the very first things I do when I start working with a nutrition client or group of clients is take them through a mindful eating exercise. It involves a series of questions encouraging people to use their senses to explore food before eating it. The purpose of the exercise is not to categorize food as 'good or bad' but look at how people are eating and the feelings that often emerge while they're eating. Every single person I've led through this experience has had at least one takeaway. Experiences range from basic awareness about food to very profound feelings and ideas around eating. It's a great way to help you reflect on your habits, tastes, and associations around food.

Far too many people eat on the run; eat quickly; eat standing up, ready to move onto the next task, instead of sitting to enjoy their meal. They distract themselves while eating which results in eating too little, or in most cases, too much. These behaviours lead to a disconnection with food; feelings of guilt and shame; overeating, binge eating, addictive eating, stress eating, and difficulty overcoming food cravings. Life circumstances can make it challenging to be still and focus on eating your food. However, when you do, you develop a positive relationship and habit around the act of eating.

Here are my favourite ways to encourage *mindful eating*:

- Pick one meal each day that you and your family can enjoy together without distraction – no phones, no devices, and no TV. Simply sit together, converse, laugh, show appreciation to the cook and the food, and simply be.
- Put your fork down between bites. Savour the taste and texture of food.
- Take a breath every few bites to help you slow down and be more mindful.
- Do not eat on the run. Take a few minutes to sit and eat.
- Chew your food. It takes an average of 32 chews to break

down most food. Obviously certain foods are more watery and take less effort. But for the most part, each bite should take you 30 seconds or more to chew and swallow.
- Tune into how the meal you're eating is making you feel.

Eating with mindfulness does not always mean eating slowly, nor is it something you need to do at every meal. But when you take the time to slow down and appreciate your food, you are less likely to struggle with a weight problem, indigestion, and erratic eating patterns. The more in tune with your body you become, the better you will feel, and better able to find pleasure and show gratitude for your food.

Eating mindfully is taking the time to appreciate, experience, and enjoy your food.

IN CONCLUSION

Healthy eating habits are learned and practiced. You have the ability to change old patterns that will improve your relationship with food and your nutrition through things like eating portions appropriate to your body's needs; slowing down and eating more mindfully; counting the things that matter and letting go of the rest; and of course, making sustainable choices for life. The biggest take-home message here is that it's okay to enjoy everything in moderation. Small changes to your eating habits over time will add up to a huge impact on your well-being. Don't change everything all at once. Small steps equal big success.

THE SUCCESS OF SUSTAINABLE NUTRITION

Leo's Story

The very first time I spoke to Leo, he expressed his reservations about working with a nutrition coach because of some negative past experiences. However, his daughter had given me a stellar review, so he was willing to give my coaching a shot in hopes of changing some bad habits and losing weight.

On our initial consultation call, I asked Leo what his main reservations were about hiring a coach. He said that he assumed all nutrition coaches took a similar approach that included tedious food logging, food rules, and meal plans. He did not want to count calories, do daily food journals, track things in an app, or do anything else that was too time-consuming or restrictive. He wanted simple, sustainable tools that would help him, long term. I was stoked – Leo was talking my language!

Leo told me he wanted to make a change in his eating and overall health because of what someone encouraged him to do, rather than what someone told him to do. In my opinion, being a good coach means guiding clients to their own realizations of what has to happen, not dictating or forcing people there. It's listening to their individual needs, desires, and wants. Leo was the captain of the ship and I was the pilot keeping him on course. I simply supported and guided him along the path. Ultimately, he decided what needed to happen, and did it.

We met every two weeks to check-in, set new goals, reframe negative thought patterns, and to help him make new choices. He had an idea of what he wanted to achieve and appreciated the accountability and guidance I supplied about where to start, how to make changes stick, and how to enjoy food and family gatherings without guilt or fear. Those were the tools he felt had been missing from his toolkit.

In order to deliver good coaching, there were a few key tasks that I thought he might resist. A food diary was the first. I promised that I would occasionally ask him to track his food intake over a three-day period, but for information purposes only. That's it, that's all. He understood my reasoning and agreed to send me pics of everything he consumed when asked to do so. I couldn't help him change eating habits and daily patterns that I couldn't see.

After receiving his initial food diary, we hopped on our second coaching call and went over everything in detail together. We then made a plan to clean up some of his eating habits. First, we tackled the ones that would have the biggest impact on his waist-line and overall health. Top of the list was Leo's daily dose of Diet Coke. He told me that he drank it because it was a habit, not because he loved it or felt he even really 'needed' it. It had been something he had done every day for many years without think-ing. Some concerned friends and family members challenged his choice and some even told him to stop drinking it. At the time he didn't see the downside and was unmotivated to change.

As a side note, Leo has a very 'black and white' personality. He's either in or he's out – no gray areas. There was no happy medium with his Coke habit. If he was going to kick the habit, he knew it had to be a clean break, and it had to be on his terms.

You want to know something interesting? After that food-diary call, Leo never touched another Diet Coke. It wasn't because I told him to stop, but because he no longer wanted it. He no longer saw the benefit or enjoyment and realized if he stopped, he would find enjoyment in other things and he was ready to embrace that. I made several other suggestions around the Coke but none were worth entertaining. I was impressed and to be honest, so was he.

Leo and I coached together for over eight months and he never ever reverted to his old habit. That was the first and most signifi-cant change he made, in a long list that followed. Some of his wins were less evening snacking, listening to hunger cues, not overeating, and mindful eating. He also learned to enjoy holiday indulgences and dinner parties with family and friends, while feeling fully capable of steering the ship right back on course thereafter.

Leo shared something with me that I've been told by most, if not all of my clients: 'From day one what I really like and dislike about you and your coaching style is that you really get into my head. I hear your voice encouraging me to make better choices. I hear your voice reminding me of my goals and weekly focuses. I like that you're "with me" even when you're not.'

Leo made changes for a lifetime, not a short time, and is still reaping the reward. He even signed on to work with me on his fitness and became inspired to return to weight lifting, something he enjoyed years previous. In the end, Leo lost weight, gained strength, reduced his blood pressure, and learned to be more mindful of his choices. His life changed for the better because he decided it was time and he made the effort to take action. Even at the age of 70, change is possible if you want it and if you choose it.

5

MINDFULNESS

To practice mindfulness simply means to practice full presence. It stems from Buddhist teachings and is a way to strengthen the power of your mind. Practicing mindfulness does not mean you're a Buddhist; it means you're dedicated to developing your ability to live in the present moment. It's the act of fully attending to what is happening, what you're doing, and to the space you're moving through.

The mind is so powerful that, unless you practice the skill of being present, you will easily find yourself obsessing about something that happened yesterday or fretting about what might happen tomorrow. By regularly engaging in mindful exercises, you develop the ability to react effectively when stressful situations occur, instead of finding yourself overwhelmed. This ability may be beneficial to all aspects of your life and well-being.

The best part is that each and every person has a built-in mindfulness program. Anyone, anywhere can practice being mindful without changing a single thing about who they are or how they live their life. It's in us. It's part of who we are as humans and it takes many shapes and names. If it's not something that comes easily to you or that you have never tried, the first step is to learn how to access it. Like anything else, mindfulness is something you learn through practice. The more you train your mind to be in the here and now, the easier it is to live that way.

There are many great ways to practice mindfulness. Some of the more common ways are meditation, or taking brief pauses in everyday life (for example, to breathe deeply or listen to calming music), or through a combination of meditation and other activities, such as sports or yoga. More about this later.

There is no right or wrong way to practice the art of presence.

When you first introduce mindfulness exercises into your life, try to avoid fixating on the outcome. Initially the goal might be something very basic, like tuning into your breath for one minute without losing focus. The more you practice, the longer you will be able to control your mind, your thoughts, and in turn, your actions.

Shutting off your internal dialogue is the biggest hurdle, yet you can achieve it if you are willing to commit to the process. Scientific evidence and real-time experience demonstrate the positive effects of being more present. It benefits our health, happiness, stress levels, work life, and relationships.

One of the best parts of being more mindful is that it sparks innovation. It's in those moments of peace, quiet, and going within, that some of your most effective, resilient, and fulfilling ideas unfold. When they do, you are more capable of dealing with the complexities and uncertainties of life. You can better cope with stress and worry by taking effective actions rather than just reacting. Your daily mindset and outlook on life improve as a result.

WHAT IS 'MINDSET' ANYWAYS?

Before we dive too far into mindset, it is important to note how the concepts of mindfulness and mindset differ and how they overlap. Because both start with the root word 'mind', many people use them interchangeably; but they are not the same. *Mindfulness* means paying attention, being present, increasing *self-awareness**, observing your thoughts, feelings, and the world around you. *Mindset* is your set of beliefs and thought patterns. Therefore, your mindset rules your behaviours, self-talk, and attitude towards life. Adrienne Lopez of MindHeartSpace offers a great analogy. She describes 'mindset' as the books and 'mindfulness' as the bookshelf.

Let's start by taking a closer look at mindset. Your mindset includes the assumptions, methods, choices, behaviours, and tools that you hold to be true. It's what you believe and how you move through life in accordance with those beliefs. You can either carry a 'growth mindset' or a 'fixed mindset'.

Growth mindset individuals believe that they have the ability to learn and improve. To get where they want to go, they are willing and able to take action and to keep at it until they arrive. They don't back down easily. Resilience is their forte, a quality essential to creating the life you desire.

Whether the goal is to lose weight, reduce physical discomfort, or become more fit, three things will dramatically increase the likelihood of a person achieving it: the belief that they can do it; a commitment to the process; and a good support system. All three are typical of growth mindset individuals. They are willing to learn from their experiences, take action toward their goals, and persist, despite challenges, big or small.

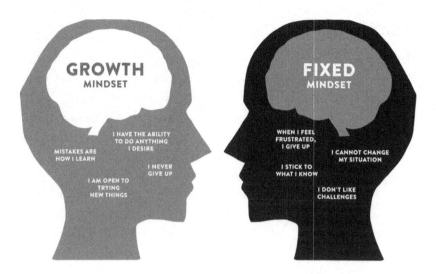

On the flip side, those who live life with a *fixed mindset* believe that their personal traits and circumstances cannot be altered. As a result, they lack the motivation to develop skills for self-improvement. Someone with a fixed mindset is much faster to pack it in or self-sabotage their efforts when things get hard. Convinced that talent alone decides a person's destiny, they are unwilling to make the effort to change their outcomes. Fixed mindset individuals also maintain that something they have tried in the past, and did not work then, never will. They confine themselves in a box without the motivation to look around for a way out.

If you are someone who struggles with a fixed mindset, the good news is that *you* have the choice to change it. Does it take time and energy? Absolutely. Does it take practice? You bet. But I promise you, it's totally worth it. Making small shifts in your thinking, being consistent, and catching yourself when you feel limited or blocked will help you move from a fixed mindset to a growth mindset. Using some of the tools and techniques I share in the *The 6 Elements of Health* downloadable workbook (see resources section), you can get started on your journey to more positive thinking and belief in yourself. Look to the Resources section at the end of this book for links.

• • •

THE VALUE OF VISUALIZATION

I had never heard the words 'mindfulness' or 'mindset' until I was almost 30. Meditation was something I thought others did and I was well into my 30's before I bothered to find out how it could benefit my life. My first experience using mindfulness and harnessing the power of my thoughts was during a Sport Psychology class. It introduced the power of visualization in relation to performance – a perfect match for a visual learner like me.

That class became one of my favourites. I found the concepts fascinating and practical, offering tangible benefits when applied in the real world. Visualization simply made sense to me; it was a tool that I wanted to use.

I began applying visualization not only to my personal life, but to my professional life. It's one thing to be physically strong, but it's another thing entirely to engage in practices that help you develop resilience, persistence, trust, and the personal conviction that anything is possible. I have always considered myself an optimistic person, who has no trouble finding the silver lining in any given situation. But this was a whole new arena and a whole new set of skills. It was a way to take my sports performance and personal life to the next level.

Trust that everything you experience in life happens for you, not to you.

My first-ever deliberate application of visualization was in softball. Picture this. My team, the Isotopes, was up against the top team in our league, vying for a spot in the season finals. It was one of the most important games of the season. I was the pitcher, and the pressure to perform was huge. If you've never played baseball, imagine a time in your life when you felt that everything was riding on you. That's how I felt.

As a pitcher, your team relies on your ability to 'manage' the opposing team, set the tone of the game, and stay focused and sharp. You have to be able to read the other players, capitalize on their weaknesses, and play the game prioritizing your team's strongest natural abilities and skill. My team and I really wanted to win that game, out of pride, but also because we knew we could.

Personally, I felt as though we had already won. Throughout that season I did one thing that I had never done in 30 years of softball. I used visualization to rehearse, plan, and prepare how my team and I would emerge victorious. In the days leading up to the season's final games, while showing up to practices, I also rehearsed everything mentally.

In my mind I planned how the ball would leave my hand, where it would hit the catcher's glove, and how fast it would go. I even knew the song I would be singing on repeat as I stood on the pitcher's mound: 'This Is What You Came For,' by Calvin Harris and Rihanna.

Nothing was going to rattle me. Nothing could shift my laser focus. I had built up my mindset muscle so that no matter what came my way, I would stand strong under pressure. I visualized striking key players out, catching line drives, and supporting my team in any way possible. I was not afraid or nervous but excited for the challenge. I arrived at that game well-prepared, regardless of the outcome.

Guess what? We won our game that night against the toughest team in our division with a score of 4-1. As I write these words, I get shivers through my body. It was powerful. It was a stellar game and I can go back to that moment in a heartbeat. I can honestly tell you that I would not have been as successful that night and many nights thereafter, without the mental practice of visualization.

At first I used visualization just for sport and athletic performance, but now it has become a daily routine. Within ten minutes of waking you will find me sitting on my yoga mat or doing some simple stretching while meditating, affirming, or using visualization to start my day, at least five days a week. It's something I can no longer live without because I see, feel, and live the benefits of it every day.

Visualization is a great tool and one that I use to increase my performance, stay in a state of positivity, and focus on my dreams. In order for this or any other mindful practice to work for you, you have to be open-minded, have faith in the process, and be willing to practice. It's a journey well worth the work.

STRENGTHENING YOUR MINDSET MUSCLE

Many simple and effective tools can help you strengthen your mindset. I just introduced you to one of those tools, *visualization*. Let me tell you more about it, and about another of my favourites, *gratitude*.

The point of visualization is to create and see in your mind what is likely to play out in your life. For example, by seeing and feeling every aspect of that softball game in just the way I wanted to play it, I was able to stay 'in my zone' when the pressure was on. It was easier to return to 'my center' and remain calm and confident because of the plan in my mind that I had rehearsed. That works for any aspect of your life that you desire to improve, not just sports.

If you can see it in your mind, you can live it in your life.

Visualizations are available on YouTube for anything and every-thing you want to improve in your life. There are visualizations to improve your health, help you heal from injury, increase your sense of calm, energize you, and help you get into a positive state of mind. Visualization is a cheap, simple, and powerful tool that will strengthen your mindset muscle.

Living in a state of gratitude is another great practice that perpet-uates positivity and optimism. When you focus on and appreciate what you already have, you attract more into your life. I'm sure you know someone who lives life with a sense of happiness and joy despite their life circumstances.

For me, it's my brother. Due to spina bifida and hydrocephalus, he has lived with both a mental and physical disability since birth.

That's placed him in a very medically fragile state. He's had more surgeries than I can count, beat the odds for survival more times than a cat with nine lives, and endured more challenges than anyone I know. But, on any given day, I can ring him and he's almost always 'great', no matter how many needles he's been poked with, how long he's had to wait for the HandyDart, or anything else that may have occurred.

He lives his life in the moment and in a state of positivity, accepting and grateful for what is. Yet if anyone could justifiably say 'screw it' and throw in the towel, it's him.

The thing is, we cannot be in a state of gratitude and in a state of want at the same time. When you focus on the good things in your life, you start to crowd out the not-so-good things.

I encourage you to take a moment right now and say aloud the five things you are grateful for. Go ahead!

Now try and make gratitude a habit. Come up with five things to be thankful for each day: the fresh air, clean water, great conversa-tions, family you can count on, clothes on your back, food on your table, jobs that pay the bills, friends, family, love, support, and so on. Everything counts. Nothing is too small to be thankful for.

Gratitude is a state of being, not just a 'cool idea' to do once and forget.

MORNINGS ARE SACRED

I remember my alarm going off at 5:30 am for weeks on end. It wasn't my first choice, but it's what I thought I 'needed' to do. I rolled out of bed, grabbed a glass of water, and hit the 'on' button of the computer. As the wheel spun and the programs loaded I sat there, my eyes barely open and still crusted with sleep, trying to wake up. I got out of bed early each morning with big plans for a productive day. I had set deadlines for myself, my business, and made a to-do list as long as my arm, and I was going to be successful, damn it!

What I didn't realize, and what I learned years later, was that our brains require anywhere from 30 to 60 minutes to actually wake up, power up, and prepare for the day. Rolling out of bed and right onto the computer was not efficient or recommended. In fact, it was one of the last things I should have been doing if I wanted to set myself up for success.

Thanks to Mel Robbins and her book, *The 5 Second Rule*, I began to create a new set of morning routines. She taught me to value my mornings and how important it is to really prepare myself and my mind for the day. The book is chock-full of great teachings to which I constantly refer. It's led me to practices that have not only helped me, they have stuck with me. (One more item on my list of things to be grateful for.)

One of the biggest takeaways was that whatever we choose to do in the first 30-60 minutes after waking sets the tone for the entire day ahead. This was a wake-up call. Waking up half asleep, trying to be productive and inspiring while responding to emails, fielding client needs, and writing engaging and effective marketing posts were not the way I should have been starting my day.

It took time to change my habits, but the more I did, the better I felt and more positive and productive I became. Upon waking, I started spending the first 30 minutes with a cup of tea, enjoying the quiet of the house, and meditating or reciting positive affirmations while stretching or doing some light exercise. I consciously made the choice to stop diving directly into pressure and productivity. Instead, I use those first 30 minutes as time to set my mind up with feelings of calmness and abundance and with positive thoughts.

This one small shift in my mindset and my routines has had an enormous impact on my life and my career. I chose how I wanted to live my life and what I wanted to feed my brain each and every morning. We can choose to wake in chaos and stress, jump on the computer, and run around the house getting ready for work or the kids off to school. We can even choose to hit snooze three times, so we're having to run harder and faster than ever.

Alternatively, we can choose to get up a few minutes before everyone else. Then, basking in the peace and quiet, we can plan how we want the day to roll out, and allow our brains to slowly wake and prepare for whatever that day brings.

How are you starting your day? Is there room for improvement? Start with small steps that will take you closer to your desired feelings, and choose to make your mornings sacred. What do you really have to lose?

BUILD YOUR SELF-AWARENESS

To have *self-awareness* means you know and understand your own character, feelings, motives, and desires. You have the ability to recognize yourself as an individual separate from the people and environment around you. People possess self-awareness in two ways: externally and internally.

Your level of personal awareness differs from one area of your life to another. *External self-awareness,* as it relates to health and well-being, refers to your ability to direct your focus through proprioception (external means). This is a fancy way of explaining how you focus your awareness on the movement and sensations of your muscles and joints. It also relates to the awareness you have beyond the body itself, in regard to your posture, body positioning, and balance as you move about your day.

Internal self-awareness concerns the sensations inside your body that you notice through interoception (internal means). This includes things like a fluttering heartbeat, the pace of your breath, lung pain from cold weather, the urge to use the washroom, hunger, and satiety.

You are self-aware when you have a strong sense of who you are, your strengths, weaknesses, thoughts, beliefs, emotions, and motivations. The more self-aware you are, the easier it is to understand others and their perceptions of you. Without self-awareness, it's easy to do things in your life without much thought. When it comes to health and well-being, it's important that you tune into your body's needs, sensations, what feels good or bad, and what brings you pleasure. That's your body's way of giving feedback, and without this feedback we are unable to improve, change, and grow.

Greater self-awareness means you are less likely to do things like skip lunch break, eat foods that aggravate your digestive system, eat meals on the run, and drink copious amounts of coffee instead of getting more sleep. You are less likely to neglect your physical body, by stretching to the point of pain, exercising too aggressively for your skill level, or doing things to the point of injury.

In order to improve your self-awareness, there are many things you can do. Daily self-reflection is a good place to start. This usually means taking five or ten minutes at the end of your day to think about how you felt, how you performed at work or for sport, how you handled stressful situations, how your body feels, and what you could do differently, given the same circumstances next time. Self-reflection is simply looking at yourself as if in a mirror and describing what you see. In this particular exercise what you want to do is take a moment to think about how you acted, reacted, and what motivated you to do what you did. Many people find this practice easier and more effective through journal writing, to fully self-reflect on the page. But if you prefer to sit and think, go for it!

Show gratitude for what you have and it will bring you closer to what you want.

Meditation is another way to increase self-awareness. If you're someone who struggles with meditation, before you skip this section all together, hear me out. I am not someone who sits still for long periods of time nor can I easily 'shut off' my brain as meditation requires. Meditation was fine for others, I always thought, but never 'for me'. Like many other things I tried in life, it did not come easy, but the more I practiced, the easier and more beneficial I found it. After two years of consistent practice, dropping into a quiet, meditative space has become a way of life. It's how I start most days and it sets the tone for the day ahead.

Anyone who uses meditation or has tried to implement this practice knows that the mind is the biggest obstacle standing between you and your self-awareness. But with practice, meditation allows you to activate different centers in your brain and move between high and low frequencies (or states of being). It provides more opportunity to choose your thoughts and the subject or issue on which you wish to focus.

There is no right or wrong way to meditate. You don't have to sit cross-legged on a cushion with your palms up and your eyes closed, but you can. The goal is to find what works for you and do it.

There are two ways I enjoy meditation. The first is more traditional. I enjoy sitting on my yoga mat crossed-legged, with tall posture, palms on my knees (facing down), and following along with a guided visualization or breathing meditation. The second way is listening to an 'I AM' affirmation meditation while stretching or doing yoga. There is something about the slow methodical movement of my body while reciting the affirmations that takes me to a positive place and helps me stay focused on the present moment. Visualization or affirmation-style meditations can be extremely helpful if you find your mind wanders. This will give you a focus as well as help to guide your thoughts. You will find a great beginners' visualization and meditation bundle in the Resources Section of this book. Starting with a five-minute meditation and then building on that will help set you up for success.

If you're someone who finds it impossible to make or take the time to sit quietly in the morning, a walking meditation may be helpful. It allows you to move about your day while being guided with calming music, deep breathing, or specific actions to create more mindfulness. It's a great way to help clear your mind and create a sense of peace in your heart. Or, sometimes you just need some simple calming music in conjunction with deep breathing. Whichever way you choose to use to meditate, they all are powerful: they can alter your state of being for the better.

MINDFUL LIFE LESSONS

Lesson #1

We sat on the porch sipping raspberry yogurt smoothies, looking across the freshly-cut yard, the gardens, the flowers, and taking in the cool summer breeze. It was a perfect day in so many ways. My mother-in-law, my son, and I got into a conversation about what living in a state of gratitude and abundance really means. As you can imagine, conversing with a six-year-old on a topic like this was informative, to say the least, for both him and for us.

My mother-in-law and I agreed that when you acknowledge the beauty, love, joy, and positivity that surround you, you live in a higher vibration and you feel rich. It's a 'bank account', but of valuables never found in the bank. We also agreed that *we* get to decide how we feel about what's in our bank account and, in turn, in our lives.

My mother-in-law made a comment about being rich. Up to that point my son had not contributed to the conversation, but we knew he was listening. Suddenly he chimed in, his eyes as wide as saucers, 'So, you have lots and lots of money, Granny?!' 'No,' she replied, 'I don't. But I have enough money and I am rich because I have enough of everything I need. I feel rich and that is why I'm rich.' She saw the look of confusion on his face, so she continued. 'I have a lot of love in my life, a beautiful garden, a nice home, successful and happy kids, a loving partner, and wonderful grandson. [The list went on.] The money I do have and the things in my life make me feel rich, even if others don't see it that way.'

My son turned to me, still looking quite puzzled, and asked the same question, 'Mimi, are you rich?' I replied, 'I am abundant and I feel rich in many ways, but I do not have millions of dollars, if that's what you are asking.'

After I answered his question, he let it go, but still seemed slightly confused at how we could be 'rich' without being 'rich'. It was a fantastic teaching and learning moment for all. If anything came from the conversation, I think he got the point that money is only a part of the equation and not everything. I learned that shaping his view of what really matters in life starts now. There is so much to be grateful for and so many things, apart from cash, that bring abundance to our lives. I am grateful for that conversation and that my son witnessed and took part in it.

Lesson #2

Another important life lesson and way to strengthen your mindset muscle is by realizing how much you can learn from your mistakes. Mistakes, mishaps, or unfortunate things are going to happen that simply cannot be anticipated. That's just how life works. Taking a moment to reflect on your mistakes before immediately jumping to self-criticism will help to uncover the life lesson you were supposed to learn. There is something to be gained and learned from every situation.

Instead of asking 'Why me?' after something goes badly wrong, pose yourself a simple question, like 'What was I supposed to learn from this experience?' Instead of saying, 'Of course, things like this always happen to me,' ask, 'How can I move forward with what I now know?' Mistakes are a great way to gain feedback and move forward even more energetically and resiliently than before. Learning from mistakes helps bring you back to a positive state of mind and helps you learn and improve as a person.

Mistakes are inevitable, they build resilience, and they're our greatest teachers.

I will never forget the first client I ever fitness-trained. My supervisor, who needed to make room in her schedule for other work, passed her along. I needed clientele. Unfortunately, fresh out of college, I lacked the confidence and knowledge to coach this person well. As I often do, I put on a brave face and off I went, heart pounding and palms sweating.

I felt nervous and inadequate because I did not know how to progress her exercises correctly. She had hurt her shoulder, and I was extremely concerned I would make the injury worse. It made for some very boring and basic training sessions. She never reached her weight loss goal and I felt totally defeated. I had spent several years educating myself in kinesiology and fitness, but the practical application, as I eventually discovered, would take years to master.

Looking back, I'm grateful for that experience and for the mistakes I made, regardless of how uncomfortable I felt. I would never have grown as a coach or fitness trainer had I not gone through those early challenges and experiences. I could have easily given up, but I never did. Instead, I chose to watch other, more skilled trainers, read books, and take courses that helped me gain expertise and confidence.

I knew deep in my heart that I could do better. Now, I look back and cringe at those first six months in that gym. I wished I 'knew it all' the moment my feet hit the training floor, but that's not how life works. What I got from that entry to the world of personal training was a lot of mini-failures. They provided me with the feedback I needed to get better at my craft. Feedback is what shaped me into the coach I am today. Mistakes are simply feed-back along the path to greatness.

Lesson #3

This learning experience came from working with a client named Lana. One of the first things Lana and I dove into during our time coaching together was self-love. Lana was struggling with her body image and personal belief around her self-image and beauty. She didn't feel beautiful. In her words, she had 'let herself go' in an effort to care for children and her family. She had lost her sense of self and in turn felt poorly about her physical shape. These deep-rooted feelings led to some negative internal beliefs.

In an effort to help Lana change some of the stories she was carrying, we began using body-positive affirmations. Affirmations are a great way to shift negative thoughts and feelings into positive ones. It's a way to reprogram your brain through repetition and daily practice.

If you are someone who struggles with positive self-talk, this can be a game changer. It is far healthier to recite affirmations to your-self, like 'I am strong', 'I am healthy', 'I am exactly where I am supposed to be', and 'I nourish my body well each day', than to repeat words of self-sabotage. They will only lead you down the rabbit hole of self-doubt.

Lana posted a list of body-positive affirmations on her bathroom mirror. The first few days she recited those affirmations were excruciating. There were tears and inner-critic back talk but each day she said them again, and each day it got a little easier. After a few weeks she could go through that list without tears. She had shifted her mindset and her belief about herself was also shifting. She started exercising more, choosing healthier foods, meditating, and spending more time in nature. She shifted aspects of her mental health that she didn't even realize needed shifting.

That list of affirmations was a life lesson worth learning. Lana now has a much better relationship with herself and her body then she did months ago. She messaged me to say that she now regularly tells herself 'she's a beautiful badass woman' with confidence, rather than losing her shit and bawling in a puddle on the floor. Mindset lesson for the win!

If shifting your thoughts is something you know you need to do, I encourage you to give affirmations a try. Once you start seeing and saying positive affirmations on a regular basis, you will start to change your mindset and the story you tell yourself. A key aspect of making affirmations work for you is that you have to believe them. You cannot just post niceties around your home that you actually do not believe or cannot get behind. Take a moment to listen to what comes out of your mouth and the thoughts that circulate in your mind. Ask yourself, would I say this to my best friend? If not, don't say it to yourself!

What you believe fuels your thoughts, and your thoughts are what drive your actions.

THE POWER OF PRESENCE

I have coached 100's of men and women since starting my career in the health and fitness industry in 2008. There is one thing I know for certain: the only way to make lasting and sustainable change is to have a clear vision of what you want and then get your mind in the game. Developing and cultivating your mindset and practicing the art of presence is the thread that connects each element of health and it's what will propel to reach your biggest boldest desires.

Have you ever tried to quit smoking, quit drinking alcohol, to change your eating habits, or do something else that takes every ounce of willpower, grit, and dedication you have? If so, you know what I'm talking about.

Helping people connect to their bigger 'why' means helping them come back to the present moment while setting up a clear vision for the future. What we do today sets us up for success tomorrow. If we are constantly in a state of future-thinking, we miss the opportunities that lead us to where we want to go.

To get connected to your 'why' try using this exercise. It's known as the '5 Whys':

1. If I asked you to tell me where you would like to be 6-12 months from now, what would you say? How do you want to feel? What do you want your life to look like? Your health? Your fitness? Your work? (or any other area of your life that you want to change)
2. Why do you want this? What purpose does it serve in your life? How will it change your life for the better if you achieve it?
3. Now go deeper. Why will this change your life/work/health/confidence?
4. Dig deeper still. Why do you think it will change your life/ work/health/confidence?
5. And finally, why?

For example, if I told you I would like to be able to do 15 unassisted chin-ups, 6-12 months from now, here are my '5 whys':

1. I want to feel as strong as I did when I was in my early 20's and could do at least 15-20 chin-ups.
2. Being able to do this will elevate my self-confidence and body confidence.
3. Achieving this will create a sense of satisfaction in knowing that with practice and consistency I can do whatever I set my mind to.
4. Being able to accomplish this goal will change the way I look at myself, my confidence, and my athletic abilities. Some days I do not feel strong, but I love it when I do, so I want to feel more of that.
5. I like it when others see me as strong and confident. Being able to do unassisted chin-ups is not easy for a female, so achieving this goal will feel very satisfying.

Therefore, my main 'why' (the thing driving what I hope to achieve) is that I want to be strong and confident. I want to feel accomplished and I want to push myself to do things that do not come easily to me.

Journaling is the best way to do this exercise. When you write down your '5 Whys', you will see the line running between your thoughts and your goals. Staying on the surface and setting an intention to lose 15 pounds is great, but why? Saying you want to train to run a marathon in six months time is a great goal, but why? Saying you want to start adding more fresh food to your life and avoid processed foods is great, but again, why? What is at the root of the desire and how will it change your life?

When we can tap into the root of what is driving us to make the changes we long to make, when moments self-doubt, hesitation, or self-sabotage pop up, we can quickly return to our 'why' and redirect our thoughts and actions. This can also help us stay present with what we need to do *today* that will support our future.

Another great way to improve your ability to remain present is to avoid multitasking. Doing multiple things at once means doing lots of things half-assed. Things like holding down a conversation with your kid while texting on your phone, or flipping back and forth between screens or different tasks on your computer instead of focusing on one thing and seeing it though.

By choosing to remain focused and present with one task at a time, you do that one thing really well. It reduces your stress, you perform better overall, and you are way more productive. I know this is a hard practice to conquer – I'm a total multitasker. But what I will share is that when I put my mind to a project or task and see it through to completion, I feel accomplished and elated.

Here's yet another way to be more present: conscious breathing. You probably never give your breathing much thought. It just happens. Nature designed us to breathe involuntarily so we could survive. But, when you do focus on your breathing, be it in moments of stress, anxiety, fear, worry, frustration, or anger, you are far more capable of returning to the present moment, staying calm, and making more rational decisions.

There's no better time than right now to give conscious breathing a try. What we practice is what becomes automatic when we need it. Here's how it works:

Step 1: Take a big deep breath in through your nose for a count of five. Inhale the air right down into your belly. Visualize your rib cage and belly expanding as if an umbrella opening.
Step 2: Hold that breath for five seconds.
Step 3: Exhale the air out your mouth to a count of five. Blow it out with purpose, as if letting all your stress deflate from your body.
Step 4: Repeat steps 1-3, four more times.

I call this little exercise the "5X5X5'. I like it because it's easy to remember, it requires very little thought, and it works. Performing it immediately calms my mind and body and better equips me to manage the situation at hand. Give it a try and see how you feel! Remind yourself that you cannot control all aspects of your life. Remind yourself that things are going to be okay, just breathe. You cannot be in a state of stress and calm at the same time. By choosing to breathe consciously, you are choosing calm.

IN CONCLUSION

Mindfulness can be learned and practiced in many different ways. There is no right or wrong method and the benefits are endless. In order to improve your ability to be mindful, it first helps to improve your self-awareness. Doing intentional things like slowing down, tuning into your body and mind, and making a practice of staying in the present moment are all great places to start. When you make mindfulness a daily practice, it has the potential to keep you in a state of positivity and calm, and reduce stress and anxiety. Mindfulness comes down to living in a state of presence, letting go of what you cannot change or what might happen down the road. The here and now is all you have, so enjoy it.

THE SUCCESS OF PRACTICED MINDFULNESS

Tara's Story

Tara is a high-energy and fun-loving elementary school teacher. She loves sports and goes to the gym at least five days a week. In the past, she had enjoyed cooking for herself and had even done some mindful practices, like meditation and journaling. In many ways she was a fit and health-conscious individual. Nevertheless, Tara had a few habits that she called the 'outliers'. She confessed to me that she had struggled with them for years and she wanted to kick them to the curb for good.

Tara initially reached out to me for coaching because certain aspects of her current life and the life she wanted to live were out of alignment. These were things that just didn't fit into her vision of herself. She had tried to change before but felt she couldn't do all on her own. The person she wanted to be did not smoke cigarettes and eat fast food. For her the two went hand in hand, which meant, if she could change one habit, the other would naturally follow.

Tara shared that she felt embarrassed about smoking, both in front of others and within herself. She never smoked at work or around her co-workers. She was a closet smoker. She would spend the time on her commute home from work 'rewarding' herself and decompressing from the day with a cigarette, despite the negative feelings associated with the habit. She would arrive home and light up another as a way to unwind. This after-work habit had become unconscious, just like brushing her teeth or making her morning coffee.

The interesting part was that, despite smoking a few cigarettes after work, her next routine was to head to the gym. She loved working out and how good it made her feel. But again, she would follow up that positive mid-evening routine by grabbing something 'quick' to eat, then heading home and having a few more smokes before bed. Although exercise and healthy eating were parts of her life and she enjoyed how they made her feel, she just could not find the motivation to do it for herself as often as she would have liked. She desperately wanted to kick her 'bad habits' and clean up her lifestyle.

On our first coaching call together, after gathering more information about Tara's life, she and I made a plan to kick those habits that no longer served her – a no-fail plan to change her habits and in turn her routines for good. As when I coached Leo (see Chapter 4), I didn't tell her what to do, instead I led her down a path to making her own decisions around what was needed for success. The plan included setting a 'smoking quit date' and meditating on what her life would look like without smoking. Her plan also involved making an appointment with a naturopathic doctor and an acupuncturist. This was to ensure she was clearing the toxins from her body as the cessation process began, and to help her resist the cravings that would inevitably arise.

Tara chose her quit date. She picked one several weeks away, to give her time to prepare both physically and mentally. Again, like Leo, Tara needed things to be black and white. She needed a clean break from the habit so she prepared for that. I encouraged her to remove all cigarette paraphernalia from her home, car, and purse in advance of the date. She also decided to have her car detailed, something she had to pay for and knew would deter her from lighting up in moments of weakness. The goal was to eliminate temptation and risk of relapse, while getting support from a team of professionals.

Tara had been here before – she had quit and then fallen back into her old ways in a moment of stress, desperation, and weakness. She knew this time was going to be different. She was committed and ready, and unlike previously, she had the tools and team in place to make it happen. Tara became more self-aware than ever before and she knew in order to kick her smoking and eating habits for good, she had to exercise as much awareness as possible.

The day came. Tara was ready. Instead of lighting up a smoke on her commute home she popped on a podcast in her freshly detailed car. Instead of going home after school, her usual routine, she hit the gym first. No room for temptation there. Instead of grabbing fast food, she had a weekly meal plan and a well-stocked fridge so she went home to cook dinner for herself and had enough leftovers for lunch the next day. Tara spent the first week after her quit date changing the routines in her life that prompted her to smoke. Was it easy? Heck no, but it was working.

She spent her evenings writing and spending time with family or non-smoking friends. She booked appointments for *self-care* that took up her time and made her feel her best. Anytime she felt tempted to smoke or had a pang of craving, she did some deep breathing, listened to a meditation, wrote in her journal, or went for a walk, a no-fail plan to change her habits and in turn her routines for good.

Six months after Tara's quit date, I contacted her to see how things were going. She was still a non-smoker living a healthier and happier life and she did it on her own terms, in her own way, using mindfulness and self-awareness. She didn't use patches, gums, or medication. Not that these are bad options, but you have to do what's right for you, and Tara needed to go 'cold turkey'. She also utilized the support of professionals to build her mindset, self-awareness, self-love, and resilience, something she continues to work on to this day. She has kept up regular visits to her naturopath and acupuncturist for continued support and self-care.

The question always remains, will she relapse? The truth is, 'maybe'. Anything is possible. But, a few things are certain: she has more tools at her disposal than ever before, her level of self-awareness has improved, and she has more belief in herself then she did previously. Definitely a feat worth celebrating!

6

SELF-LOVE

*S*elf-love is the sixth element of health. It also happens to be the final one that fell into place while I was organizing my ideas for this book. As I reflected on my own health journey and my education, I realized what an important role body image and self-love plays in our physical, emotional, and mental well-being. Were I to fail to give it the attention it deserves, I would be doing my clients, you the reader, and myself a disservice. Each and every choice we make to improve or change our health is stimulated by, you guessed it, self-love.

The importance to health of rest, movement, connection, nutrition, and mindfulness are, in many ways, obvious. They are the foundation for how I live, why I educate, and what I coach. But something still seemed to be missing. It was in my blind spot – right under my nose! The very thing that poses us the greatest challenge is the very thing we need most. Consequently, this chapter has been the most difficult for me to write.

As I will share with you shortly, self-love has not always been one of my strong points. Like many people, I have no problem lifting others up, helping them see the good in their minds, their choices, and their bodies. It's a lot easier for me to coach others in finding acceptance and self-confidence than to coach myself.

You've heard the phrase 'we are our own worst critics.' Although my inner critic has come a looonnnng way, there is still more work to be done. Since acknowledgment is the first step to making change, here we go, taking a deep dive into creating more self-love in our lives.

BODY IMAGE DEFINED

I'm someone who appreciates having a word or expression defined, so I can use it to make sense of the world. I appreciate clarity, and definitions provide that. I know this is my truth because I lived the first 20 years of my life feeling confused and yearning to make sense of who I was and what it meant. Definitions are a way to accumulate information, reflect on it, and then decide what it will mean to you and your life. That is why I decided to include Kristy's Health Definitions in the additional resources section at the back of the book. They are words that I perceive to be important to my life, and the meanings I have chosen to give them.

Body image happens to be one of those expressions. Let's take a closer look at it and how it relates to beauty.

The *Merriam-Webster Dictionary* defines 'body image' as a subjective picture of one's own physical appearance, established both by self-observation and by noting the reactions of others.

The *Oxford Learner's Dictionaries* say 'body image' is a person's mental picture of their physical appearance and how good or bad it is, especially in comparison with how they think they should look. It then uses the words in a sentence: 'Young girls can struggle with their own body image as a result of seeing perfect photos of celebrities.' It also talks about how social media can have a negative influence on how people perceive their bodies and promote an unrealistic body image.

Finally, the National Eating Disorder Association defines 'body image' as how you see yourself when you look in the mirror or when you picture yourself in your mind. It encompasses what you believe about your appearance, how you feel about your body based on things like your height, shape, and weight and how you sense and control your body as you move.

From each of these definitions it is clear that body image is how we feel about ourselves, the way we compare ourselves to others, and how we 'measure up' to the standards that have been set for us by society. There is no single 'correct' body image, and that's liberating. We get to choose how we define our bodies and how we imagine ourselves to look. We get to choose what matters most to us and live by the standards we set for ourselves.

From their earliest years, so many girls and women internalize the messages from movies, social media, peers, and from our families. These messages can either lead to positive or negative ideas about our bodies and body image. The development of a healthy body image is important for overall well-being and the prevention of things like disordered eating or eating disorders.

I encourage you to take a moment and define your body image for yourself. What comes to mind when you think about your own body image? How do you want others to feel and define themselves?

I define body image as the perception we carry about ourselves, how others view us, and how we view them. I believe that how we perceive our looks, the way we walk, talk, and carry ourselves, are all things that we project into the world around us. I also believe that confidence-boosting exercises, seeking out positive role models, surrounding ourselves with people who uplift us, and staying true to ourselves, will have a positive impact on our body image.

The good news is that no matter what age or stage you're at, there is always room for self-improvement and this includes improving your body image. Just like practicing *body neutrality**, choosing self-love over self-sabotage is the very first step. Changing negative thought patterns and feelings into positive ones is not going to happen overnight, but like anything in life, practice leads to change for the better. Changing the pattern changes the way you feel and eventually your level of self-acceptance.

We are unable to focus on both positive and negative thoughts and feelings at the same time. It's not possible. When you focus on the positive, you crowd out the negative. You get to choose what you give energy to each day, whether that be your body image or something else. That's powerful.

A RECENT HISTORY OF BODY IMAGE

I've never been much of a history buff. In fact, I just barely passed (the mandatory) Grade 9 high school history class, and have never pursued the matter since. But, like many things, whether or not you enjoy a subject is more about how it is taught than about the subject matter itself.

For example, while I was researching 'body image', a lot of interesting information came up on beauty 'ideals' and the history of body image and beauty. Learning where we've come from helps us understand where we are today, and how we got here. When it comes to how people approach beauty and body image, the common thread from the past to the present has been one of constant change. Some might argue that 'ideal' body images for men have changed even more drastically than those for women. Let's take a look at what has changed just over the past 150 years.

Victorian Era (late 1800's-early 1900's)

Ideal Body Images for Women
'Beautiful' women were slender and tall with a voluptuous bust and wide hips. This very incongruent look was achieved by corseting so the waist was cinched tight. What an uncomfortable way to live!

Ideal Body Images for Men

Big bellies! Men who carried more fat around the middle were considered more attractive than thin ones as fat signified wealth. There were even Fat Men's Clubs because a man's weight equated to his status.

This was the last era where having a big belly was viewed as attractive and it's a good thing, too. The risk for cardiovascular disease is in direct correlation to carrying too much abdominal weight.

1920's

Ideal Body Images for Women

Beauty ideals for women had changed quite drastically by the 'Roaring 20's'. Now women were considered 'beautiful' if they were flat-chested, with boyish figures.

There was also an 'epidemic of eating disorders' during this time period. They resurged in the 1980's, and in fact typify periods of history in which the ideal image of women was comparatively thin.

Ideal Body Images for Men

Standards of men's beauty had also changed by the 1920's. Hollywood films were becoming popular, and the camera made people look 20 pounds heavier. So on the one hand, there was pressure on men to stay thin. On the other hand, the muscular, dashing figures of movie stars became all the rage.

1950's

Ideal Body Images for Women

Here now was the golden era of Hollywood. Marilyn Monroe took the spotlight. Her voluptuous 35-22-35 inch figure was the pinnacle of beauty, despite the fact that she was two or three inches larger than most American women of the time.

Besides being a civil rights activist, Monroe was sexual in ways that others were not during this time in history.

Ideal Body Images for Men
For men, beauty ideals had shifted slightly from those of the 40's. The 'executive look' was now in vogue. It was less about looking strong and more about having a trim waist, broad shoulders, and tall build.

1960's

Ideal Body Images for Women
The sexual revolution triggered a significant reversal in a woman's idealized image. Being thin and androgynous was the rage, witness 'Twiggy', a supermodel with a flat chest, short hair, slight frame, and boyish look. This was significantly different from Monroe's famous look, just a decade earlier.

Ideal Body Images for Men
Men either embraced the corporate world, wearing clean, well-cut suits, or went 'bohemian', by assuming the non-conformist look of artists.
Instead of cut abs and chiseled arms, the beauty of the male physique was measured in terms of how trim it was and the amount of chest hair. The more the better!

1970's

Ideal Body Images for Women
Women's beauty was about looking svelte and curvy like a

supermodel. It was the era of disco, slim hips, and flat stomachs.

This was also the time when anorexia was getting mainstream coverage and the use of diet pills was on the rise.

Ideal Body Images for Men

For men, beauty was all about androgyny. Guys like Mick Jagger and David Bowie set a gender-bending body image on stage, causing the period to be named 'Maccioni's', after a swanky Italian restaurateur.

Their thin, linky frames and mixing of feminine and masculine clothing choices fascinated a large part of the population. But other stars sported moustaches and the famous bell-bottom pants.

1980's

Ideal Body Images for Women

The mainstream look for women was thin and more androgynous. But the strong, athletic, and toned female body image had also emerged.

This was the 'Supermodel' Era. Hardbodies were the rage and tall, leggy women like Cindy Crawford, Claudia Schiffer, and Naomi Campbell became household names.

Ideal Body Images for Men

The ideal male body went in very different directions. Some embraced the hard-bodied look of previous decades, now updated by Arnold Swartzenegger and Sylvester Stalone.

Hitting the gym was a sign of masculinity and the 'return to values' proclaimed by U.S. President Ronald Reagan.

Others embraced the rise of glam metal, with high-volume hair and exaggerated dress. It was time when song lyrics showcased a lust for the opposite sex and challenged thinking on gender, sexuality, and authenticity.

For the first time in history, men reported the experience of body-shaming, something that women had been dealing with for generations.

1990's

Ideal Body Images for Women

TV sex symbols like *Baywatch*'s Pamela Anderson indicate that skinny-fit with big breasts was the goal. Contrast that with beauty ideals in the fashion industry, which reverted to the "skinny heroin chic" seen in the 60's. (Think Kate Moss, also known as the 'waif'.)

Interestingly enough, it was at this time that anorexia nervosa became the most widely-diagnosed eating and mental health disorder in history, while at the same time the World Health Organization was seeing a rise in obesity.

Ideal Body Images for Men

Ideals of the male body became even more extreme. As more superhero movies went mainstream, so did the pressure for men to look muscular and cut.

2000's

Ideal Body Images for Women

Dieting and eating disorders continued to rise as the ideal body image for women came to include tanned skin as well as (yet another unrealistic expectation) visible abs.

Ideal Body Images for Men

More action movies and superheroes continued to idolize the chiseled and cut body image for men. Many men reported feeling more anxious about their bodies than five years previous.

2010

Ideal Body Images for Women

Although an athletic body type was still the rage, the ideal female landscape shifted yet again, to focus not only on a fit body, but the size of her 'booty' (i.e., butt).

Ideal Body Images for Men

The masculine ideal has remained almost the same since the 80's, celebrating muscles and cut bodies.

Something else that has remained constant since the beginning of time is men's hair. A full head of hair has always been a beauty ideal.

Present Day

Ideal Body Images for Women

Western beauty for women in this day and age continues to be all about big butts, a flat stomach, and a slim body. But something else quite interesting and refreshing has happened: there has been a conscious shift in the way beauty is seen and our self-acceptance around it. The idea of 'body neutrality' is gaining momentum. (See below.)

Ideal Body Images for Men

The ideal male physique continues to focus on achieving a cut, muscular, and fit look.

You can see how, over time, some things have changed while how others have repeated or remained the same. You can also see that being thin is more of a modern standard. While slim, fit, and muscular describe what is considered the 'ideal' body type of the 21st century, obesity is on the rise, as is the number of people struggling to maintain a healthy body weight. As this book emphasizes, many factors contribute to a person's overall body weight, figure, and health.

Some very inspiring and reassuring research in this regard has given rise to a movement called *body neutrality**, a term coined by Green Mountain at Fox Run, in Vermont. It's a community designed for women who struggle with weight, and emotional and binge eating. The mission of the movement is to help people slowly start to strip away feelings of not being good enough, beautiful enough, or unable to measure up to the ideals of modern society. Body neutrality helps you become more gentle and kind about the way your body looks, instead of becoming obsessed with body image, which, in combination with society's expectations, provokes negative emotions in many people.

Body neutrality is a way of talking about and living in your body that encourages you to celebrate who you are and what you bring to the world, both physically and mentally. It's about marveling at how you think, what you create, and how your work and your play contribute to the world. Body neutrality is also a methodology. The time and energy spent obsessing over your body are liberated and focused instead on caring for it. Living in this way turns body image into a source of freedom and joy.

Developing a more positive body image and greater body neutrality involves shifting your mindset away from 'beauty' and towards 'health'. That old saying, 'beauty is only skin deep' is good to keep in mind. When you are healthy (or unhealthy), it affects everything else in your life, your looks and your physical body included.

Here are some ways to shift your mindset toward greater body neutrality:

- Be observant of your **self-talk**. Before speaking unkindly about yourself or others, catch yourself and reframe your thoughts into something positive.
- **Let go** of whatever does not serve you. Belittling yourself does not make the situation better. Affirm that you deserve better and give that to yourself instead.
- Write out your favourite **affirmations** on post-it notes and put them up around your home. Or pick up some affirmation cards that resonate with you. By constantly feeding your brain positive words and phrases, you will start to crowd out the negatives.
- Choose **whole foods and move your body** each day. By respecting the link between your physical and mental well-being, you can go from down in the dumps to energized and happy.
- **Get support** if you need it. Friends, family members, and counselors are great options.
- **Be patient** with yourself. Changing a lifetime of negative thoughts will take time and effort. Be kind to yourself and your process.

This new way of thinking and acting does not mean that suddenly you will wake up in love with your body. But over time, it provides a way to generate more awareness and neutral feelings for the body you're in, and less judgment and obsession.

The concept of body neutrality is a big win in my world. Coming to a place of self-acceptance and body confidence has been something I have worked to achieve for most of my adult life. I'm still working on it. Taking an entirely different approach to my body image and what makes me beautiful has been a game changer.

If there is anything I hope you take from this book, it's this: despite what others may say or think, health is not measured by standards of weight, height, body mass index, or body figure. Health comes in all shapes and sizes and always will. I encourage you to make appreciation and self-love the North Star for your life's journey, and the practice of body neutrality your first step.

SELF ACCEPTANCE

In my late teens and early 20's I longed to find self-acceptance not only with my body image but my sexual orientation. My relationship with food and exercise were intertwined with my relationship to myself. I struggled to understand what it all meant, who I was, and how to move forward with a greater sense of confidence and self-esteem.

For the most part, I have healed my relationship with food and eating. I have learned to listen to my body's physical needs around exercise. Even though sleep has always been a top priority for me, even my sleep habits have improved, further enhancing my rest and recovery. I have successfully taught myself the art of mindfulness using meditation, affirmations, and the power of the present moment. As difficult as that can be some days, it is absolutely worth it.

And finally, I have grown more connected to my family and friends than ever before. I put a large amount of value on the family evening meal with my wife and son. A long-distance phone call to hear my mom or a sibling's voice, or a gathering in my home with family and friends – these too bring so much joy to my life.

Yet self-love has not kept pace with the rest. It's the *element** that continues to test me the most. Looking back, it's the area of my life that I always have found the most challenging.

As explained in Chapter 4, my breaking point around nutrition came in the form of an eating disorder. It reared its ugly head at a time when I felt nothing in my world was in my control. I resorted to controlling what I could. Never once during those two years did

I ever feel like I was doing the right thing. But I lacked the courage *and the self-love* to choose a new path.

Was anything to be learned from this long, dark, depressing spiral? A lot, actually. I realized that the things I was doing gained me acceptance and love from nobody, least of all from myself. I was insecure in my body, my lifestyle, and with my thoughts, yet did not know how to do differently.

Self-acceptance is a journey of deeper understanding and personal satisfaction.

Coming to a place of self-love is not narcissistic or conceited. It's having compassion, understanding, and a genuine sense of pride in who you are, what you like, how you care for your body, and what you bring to the world. Just as you show love to others, loving yourself indicates respect, a positive self-image, and personal acceptance. Practicing and living with more self-acceptance takes work, but the work is worth the result.

Truth be told, we all have something to work on. Even when we think we don't, we do. Even when we think we have healed, let go, and moved on, things 'long gone' will trigger us and creep into our awareness. There will still be moments when we drop back into self-doubt, self-sabotaging behaviours, self-criticism, or judgment. It doesn't mean all the work we have put in is for loss or that we cannot stand in confidence. It just means that there are more layers of the onion to peel away. I'm still peeling that onion today. But it's getting smaller, and that's a win worth celebrating!

THE BEAUTY OF BURLESQUE

I can honestly say that I had never felt a strong sense of confidence or sexiness living in my half-feminine (breasts, face, butt, and hips) and half-masculine body (upper body, midsection, short edgy hairstyle, and calves) until my early 30's. It wasn't until I stepped on stage to do burlesque for the first time that something shifted in me. Something big that I had never experienced before.

What is burlesque you might ask? Well, simply put, it's a dramatic and musical style of art. Burlesque shows can be delivered in a 'variety show' format, each act as its own mini play, an over-the-top presentation of the self. It's parody at its best, and a show where you should expect the unexpected. It attracts all body types, shapes, and sizes and showcases people's flair for life through dance, music, and comedy. It's also the fastest way to get over any blocks to finding your body confidence. Typically, the cast members and audiences attracted to these shows are women and couples ready to be pushed outside their comfort zone.

Talk about being surrounded by empowered women and men flaunting everything they've got to evoke laughter, emotion, and realness. It's like nothing you have ever experienced, both as a performer and audience member. At least it was for me growing up with such a sheltered lifestyle and a prudish mom. (Sorry Mom, I love you!)

My burlesque debut was with an amazing troop of body-confident women, and it was then and there that my sense of self-love made a tremendous breakthrough. It pushed me beyond what I thought possible and it showed me that I was capable of living in my body without reservation or fear of judgment. It also forced me to not give a damn. That first performance I danced and frolicked on stage and held nothing back. Admittedly, I may have had a little help from my flask of Fireball whiskey, but my confidence came from inside of me. I showed up in the flesh and fully exposed. I even lost a pastie (the little sequins that cover your nipples) in the big finale. I felt a sense of confidence and more alive in my body and in my heart than ever before.

Your fears only have as much power as you give them.

That was not the last time I got on stage to perform. Many more routines and shows helped me build my body confidence. Without these life experiences, deep in my heart I know that I would not have arrived at where I am today.

People who have never struggled with body image or something as severe as an eating disorder do not understand what a daily internal battle others are going through. In my case, a negative internal dialogue was 'on replay' and I could not shut it down. It took up a lot of energy. Not a day went by that I didn't grapple with my deepest, darkest inner feelings and desires and feel powerless to change them.

For so many years I found myself challenged to meet the expectations of 'others'. I thought that my self-worth was in direct correlation to the way I looked, the way I carried myself, and my sexual orientation. I chose those feelings and actions because they made me feel safe. But by doing so, I brought upon myself a great deal of anxiety, digestive problems, an eating disorder, and a distorted body image. What I longed for was unconditional love and acceptance. I wanted them from others, when in reality what I needed was love and unconditional love within myself. I found my true self on that stage doing burlesque and have never looked back.

Soon after, I started exploring my self-image and my body confidence. I also started working with a counsellor, studying nutrition, and surrounding myself with people who accepted me just as I was.

By sharing, honestly and openly, the messiest and most challenging pieces of my life, I believe that I was healing myself, and in turn, helping others to heal. I began to forge a new path that provided me with hope for a healthier future.

REPROGRAM THAT INNER VOICE

There are many studies of body image and body dissatisfaction. Despite their differences, there is an overriding consensus that most men and women are dissatisfied in their bodies. According to a *Global News* article in 2015, a global survey indicated that the percentage of people aged 15 and older who struggle with overall body dissatisfaction is very high.

Although we are seeing changes (for the better) from one generation to the next, 91% of women and 87% of men continue feeling unhappy with their bodies. The article went on to explain that places like Mexico, Brazil, and Argentina had the highest rankings for body satisfaction while the Japanese, British, Russians, South Koreans, Swedes, and Australians were the most body critical. It's clear that geographic location and culture plays a role in body satisfaction.

Regardless of where surveys are done, the vast majority of people move through their lives feeling unhappy or embarrassed with the way they look. Far too many people are quick to judge, shame, feel guilty, or put themselves down. They have a video reel repeating in their mind that tells them they are too fat, too thin, too tall, too short, too wide in the hips, have too much cellulite, are too outspoken, too confident, or any other 'too' that burdens them. It's easy to succumb to that 'mean' voice but we can learn to turn down the volume on our inner criticism. I think we can do better, as a society and as individuals.

Our body image and body confidence are established from a very young age. The actions, choices, and comments of parental figures, siblings, family, and the people we hang out with all shape how we view ourselves and the world around us. These influences can have either a positive or negative effect on our entire path and outlook.

Take my client Lori, for example. After many years of putting her self-care last she was ready to change her old patterns. She wanted to build strength, improve her eating habits, and find connection with others. Most importantly, she longed to improve her self-love and self-confidence.

Within the first two weeks of working together, Lori also started my self-study program, 'Vibrantly Confident'. It's a three-part video program to help you develop more self-acceptance, make peace with your body, and turn your triggers into your triumphs. After completing the first video and accompanying exercises, Lori messaged me her truths. She was unable to get through the list of 'positive body image affirmations' without balling her eyes out. The words of people around her and from her own internal chatter had affected her so negatively that she could not recite the list of affirmations without tears. This is when you know the work you're doing is powerful and needed. (For more on 'Vibrantly Confident', see the Resources section.)

When we start peeling away the layers of deep-seated emotion and hurt that we carry about ourselves, we set ourselves free. We start embracing who we are and what we bring to the world, beyond our body image and our looks. We go so much deeper. You know something? One week later, Lori sent me another message. It said, 'I got through those affirmations today without crying. That was my win of the day.' Hearing this, I knew Lori was beginning to develop a better sense of self and beginning to find peace and love with her body.

What we see and hear is what we know. Whether they were said or we witnessed them, things get ingrained in us and only we have the ability to break the cycle. Parents who go on a new fad diet every other month, or claim their butt is getting big and they should get more exercise, or comment about how much they eat or don't eat – all these things imprint on children. How about the dance teacher who pulls us aside to say we need to lose ten pounds to make the dance company try-outs? This stuff makes me want to rebel. It's sad, but it happens. And when it does, that is when we develop a poor relationship with our bodies and with food.

From a very young age many people start to build a wall around themselves. It acts as a barrier to keep them 'safe' from comments and judgments that live outside of them. All the while, they are still internalizing every last word, comment, or unrealistic body image they encounter. They are comparing their bodies to those of others, comparing their looks, their clothes, their relationships, and their material belongings. The list goes on.

There is something else many people do not stop to consider: the many forms that body shaming can take. Almost every single woman I know carries personal insecurities and lacks body confidence. The most attractive woman you have ever met likely struggles with her body image. It's sad and unfortunate, but it's the truth and should not be downplayed. Never assume someone has it easier than you.

We all have baggage, experiences, and triggers. Something I have come to realize as a female now in mid-life is that what others think and say about me is simply a reflection of them. It's not about me at all. When I walk through the world with confidence about who I am, how I dress, the size and shape of my body, I hold the power. I decide what I will let penetrate my being, and what I let roll off.

There are a few very specific things I did to gain more body confidence. They took time and practice but each was well worth the effort. On days when I'm feeling low or down on myself, I revert back to these exercises to help shift my thoughts and my actions. I believe every single person has the ability to shift their thinking. Regardless of how you were brought up, the hurts you've felt, the things you've heard or seen, or the challenges you've faced, you get to choose a new path right now. You can change your story.

I encourage you to give any of the following simple exercises a try and see what unfolds in your life. Obviously, this list is not exhaustive, but it's what helped me love myself more, and I hope it helps you too.

- Do something you've always thought about, but felt too shy. For me it was getting on stage and performing. It happened to be in the form of burlesque but it could have been speaking or dancing too.
- Take a moment each day to remind yourself of your best qualities. Dig deep and see what you come up with.
- Wear clothes that make you feel your best. If that's a t-shirt and jeans, great! If that's a sundress and sandals, wonderful. Wear what makes you feel confident and sexy.
- Talk to a therapist you trust. I never grew up with any form of counselling but when I was in my late 20's and early 30's I would never have had the courage to deal with all the crap from my past had I not opened up to Anita. She has been a rock in my adult life and I am eternally grateful for her.
- Get rid of your scale and focus on counting the right numbers! I threw out mine and promised never to count another pound or calorie as long as I lived. That was not only empowering, but liberating. I've never looked back. (More about this, below.)

True life experience is the difference between wishing for something and actually living it.

The truth is, we all have a choice. We have a choice either to react and let the opinions and comments of others affect us, or let them roll off our backs like water. When we are reactive we give our power to others. When we are confident, centered, and true to ourselves, we take back our power.

If someone close to you throws a dig your way, makes a comment about the food you're eating or your weight, you get to choose whether or not that dig gets any energy. You can choose to ignore it and walk away. You can choose to engage, possibly argue, and defend yourself. Or you can politely say, 'I'm choosing not to let your comments affect me,' and then remove yourself from the situation. This takes practice but when the time comes and you're ready, it's pretty freaking rewarding.

WORK TO YOUR STRENGTHS

It's not too often you see a large-framed man or woman performing ballet. But if you have a larger frame and love to dance, go for it! We also don't usually see small-framed, light-weight men or women playing football or hockey. But that doesn't mean you can't. Truth be told, our body type can help or hinder our ability to perform (especially in elite sports) or even draw us to certain activities. You get to decide how you want to approach movement and exercise. But finding what your body likes most can sometimes help you find something you're not only good at, but something you will enjoy and stick with.

What I mean when I say 'work to your strengths' is just that: do the things that you enjoy and make you feel your best. The energy and pressure you put on yourself to look a certain way, lift a certain amount of weight, do something because you 'think' you should, or play a certain sport because you feel pressured – it's simply a waste, in my opinion. Focus on the great things your body can do and do them often. That is how you create more joy in movement, overall happiness, and better health.

Perhaps you are unsure of what you like to do, or have forgotten to enjoy movement. If so, begin by trying different activities and classes until you find something you enjoy. In some cases this might mean stepping outside your comfort zone and being willing to appreciate all that your body *can* do and then doing more of that.

The point is, we are no more likely to excel at all sports or physical activities than we are all destined to be great bakers, gardeners, dancers, artists, or musicians. Our bodies' physical make-up, life experiences, muscle fibres, and interests help guide us along our path. We are not hardwired to be great at everything or even to like everything we try.

We each have our own set of strengths and things that bring us happiness. The more you explore, the more likely you are to find new activities that light you up and make you feel good. With a better understanding about what your body is capable of and how you feel, it's easier to focus on the things you're good at, and pass on the rest.

BODIES ARE DIFFERENT (AND THAT'S OK)

One of the most interesting aspects of working in health and fitness is 'people watching'. Sometimes I do this unconsciously and other times, like during client consultations and assessments, deliberately. Either way, I regularly find myself assessing why a person walks the way they do and what their movement patterns say about them. Their flexibility, overall mobility, and posture are also big indicators of how a person is functioning. When you look at as many bodies in a day as I do with such focus, you start to notice things that others don't.

The other thing I find fascinating is human body types, and how body type relates to the way someone carries themselves, to their self-confidence, and to their self-love. Just like animals, humans have a blueprint. A specific number of fingers and toes, legs, arms, eyes, ears, etc. But within those parameters, there is a lot of variation. Specifically, around the type of body we inhabit. It is something over which we have very little control. We are born with a certain set of genes and although you can use food and exercise to manipulate your physique, your actual body type cannot be changed in the same way. Knowing your body type can help you navigate your body image and work to its strengths.

Body type should not be confused with the body images idolized by societies, historically and today (refer to pages 128-133 above). Comparing yourself to Marilyn Monroe or some other 'ideal body image' will not improve your self-esteem. Although the 'hourglass figure' (36-24-36 inch) exists, it is uncommon. Women's bodies come in all shapes and sizes, each of which can be desirable or attractive.

I struggled to accept my thin, lean, and lanky body type for many years. I always wanted to be more muscular and stronger. I finally came to terms with the fact that I have to cater to what I've got and accept that some things simply cannot change. That's what makes us unique, and, well, us. Embracing our bodies for exactly what they were designed to do is very liberating. Instead of being focused on bench pressing my body weight, for example (something I could do but with negative effects on my shoulders), I started to focus on my ability to master core and plyometric style exercises because of my body type.

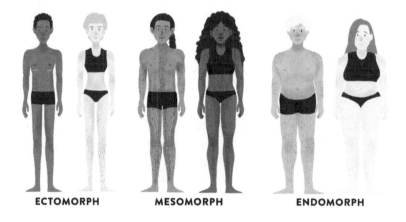

ECTOMORPH   MESOMORPH   ENDOMORPH

Base your opinion of yourself on the size of your heart, not on the size of your jeans.

Each body type comes with its own strengths, weaknesses, and nutritional requirements. For example, if you are an ectomorph like me, you tend to be lean, have longer limbs, and find it challenging to put on weight. You eat smaller meals more often, and typically thrive on a diet that includes more carbohydrates than are beneficial to other body types. This body type and shape can typically be an asset in things like swimming, soccer, marathons, biking, and activities that require speed and agility.

If you're a mesomorph, you likely have an aptitude for sports, and the ability to gain and lose weight with little effort. What suits you best is a diet with more protein and fats, and less carbs. Mesomorph body types are typically good at figure skating, gymnastics, bodybuilding, rugby, hockey, and yoga.

People with the third body type, the endomorphs, tend to put on weight easily and keep it on. They have to monitor their food portions a little more closely and do best with a balanced diet of protein, fat, and carbs. They are generally strong-boned and can build muscle quickly. This body type is not built for speed and agility like the ectomorphs, but for strength activities, like power-lifting, boxing, weight lifting, rowing, and wrestling.

A better understanding of your body type and its specific characteristics can help you choose sports or activities. Certain things will be more suited to your physique, enjoyment, and overall feeling of *success**.

This information about body types is not intended to deter you from doing sports or activities outside of what's 'typical'. I simply want you to understand that some things suit certain people better, and when we work with our strengths we are often much happier. Many people have combined characteristics from two body types and this presents opportunities to succeed at a wider range of sports and activities. We should always do what works for us, for our interests, and for our bodies, regardless of what others might say or think.

DITCH THE SCALE

Many people spend their lives chasing a number on their bathroom scale in hopes that they will find peace and contentment within themselves. For most, the scale is a source of stress, frustration, negativity, and obsession. I know this all too well. Once upon a time I also measured my self-worth, confidence, and progress by what was reflected back to me on that scale each and every day. While struggling to keep my weight at a certain number (one that I had chosen), I missed all the other amazing physical and mental gains I was making. Instead of focusing on my strength, endurance, muscle tone, energy levels, happiness, and improved self-confidence, I was caught up in one number among many others that were far more important.

In my late teens and early 20's, while determined to stay thin (and not a healthy thin) the bathroom scale became my biggest enemy. Instead of all the other results of my efforts I chose to focus on that one. As much as I hated the fact that I had given one number so much power over me, I wasn't sure how to change that.

- I could run a five kilometre race in under 27 minutes. I could have focused on that.
- I could do over 20 chin-ups in a row. I could have celebrated that.
- I could bench press my own body weight. That did not feel like enough.
- I could play just about any sport and play it well. I was quick, agile, and a natural.

- I made light of the traits that I had, and admired the ones that I lacked.

I strove constantly for more of the things at which I was 'okay', instead of shifting my focus to the things I did well.

The day came when my relationship with the scale was no longer serving me. I became more frustrated with that number than any other in my life. I became anxious and depressed, both emotions with which I had been unfamiliar up to that point. I became food obsessed in the worst possible way. I used to be a happy-go-lucky person with lots of spunk, energy, and vitality. I felt as though my obsession with the scale was sucking everything out of me but still wanted more. I had literally lost my way.

I made the choice to get rid of it. Not just tuck it away in a closet, or under the bed, but throw it into the garbage. I made the conscious choice not to use the gym scale again and rarely went to the doctor so that scale didn't pose a problem. I had decided that the number reflected back to me was not worth the emotional and physical trouble it caused.

That was a scary and liberating day, but it was worth it. I am 41 years old and the only time I ever step onto a scale is when the doctor asks me to for medical reasons. Generally, I don't even take notice of the result. Throwing away that method of measuring my self-worth and my progress has made me a happier person.

When I began coaching my client Lily, she was a scale-obsessed individual. I could totally relate and knew there was work to be done to support her in changing her ways.

The first thing Lily did every single morning upon waking was go pee, remove her PJ's, and step on the scale hoping to see the number lower than it was yesterday. She fixated on it to such a degree that the number reflected back to her could change the course of her entire day. It could lift her up as quickly as it could drag her down. She never accounted for hormone fluctuations, water retention from food she ate, or the fact that she was building muscle and strength through weight training so she could work in her barn and ride her horses that much better.

With a lot of coaching and a lot of self-discipline, Lily slowly began to make the change. She knew weighing herself every day did not build her self-confidence or self-love, but resisted replacing that habit with a better one. After shifting Lily's thinking and educating her on the power of the mind, we reduced her weigh-in from once a day to once a week. This was really, really hard at first but soon she started feeling better and seeing the result. Eventually, with further coaching and support, we reduced her weigh-in to once every two weeks. Although I wanted her to check in no more than once a month, this was too big a jump and caused Lily a lot of anxiety and stress.

All that coaching and support did not lead Lily to toss her scale outright, but they did help her shift her habits. They helped her live her life with a great sense of daily happiness instead of letting her scale dictate how she felt about herself. You have to make changes slowly and within parameters that work for you. Each and every person is hardwired a little differently and that's okay. The point is to direct as much as energy and focus as you can on the numbers that really matter – the numbers that lift you up and make you proud.

Your self-worth is never measured, but affirmed by your level of compassion, understanding, and self-love.

Does this story hold any truth for you? If so, as hard as it may seem, ditch your scale. Doing so will shift your focus from something that holds very little weight (pun intended) to something that has the capacity to change your entire outlook on life.

. . .

IN CONCLUSION

Throughout history, the expectations set out by society have taken a toll on our self-esteem and self-love. The only person who has the ability to change thought patterns, actions, and expectations to improve their self-love is you. It might not be the easiest thing you've ever done, but the work is worth it. Loving your body, your mind, your spirit, and the special gifts only you bring to this world will change how you live your life and how you treat yourself each day. Work to your strengths, surround yourself with those who lift you up, and never let anyone tell you you're not 'good enough', 'thin enough', or 'pretty enough'. You are an amazing human being just as you are.

THE SUCCESS OF GENUINE SELF-LOVE

My Story

I am one of those people who puts 110% into everything I do, my health and fitness included. I am dedicated to making healthy food choices for myself and my family. I move my body daily, enjoy my meditation practice, am very connected to my family near and far, and I have many hobbies and interests that I love.

I am always on the go and love nothing more than being outdoors, biking, hiking, doing yard work, and playing sports. I'm more active than most people I know and always have been. At some point during adolescence I began to feel the pressure of society's expectations around my choice of clothing, hairstyle, body language, and interests. I was deeply afraid that because my desires and dreams were different from those of other girls, there was something 'wrong' with me. As a result I was always hard on myself, a people pleaser, and a perfectionist. My self-confidence was low and my self-esteem suffered as a result.

From an early age I struggled to understand society's rigid ways of classifying people as masculine or feminine. I felt like I was a mix of both. I now understand, all these years later, that what I am is androgynous. Historically this led to feelings of self-doubt, confusion, and a distorted body image. I loved being lean and strong; felt 'at home' wearing 'boy's' clothes, ball caps, and getting dirty; and I expressed my independence regularly. All these traits placed me on the masculine end of the gender trait continuum.

Sadly, all this emotional turmoil led me into a state of overall lack of care and concern for my well-being. I was in need of some serious healing and self-love, body, mind, and spirit. It's hard to approve of ourselves and love ourselves completely in the face of fear, and boy did I have plenty of that. For many years I feared that I would never meet the expectations that society and my family had of me, and that I would never fit the box into which I was being forced. I also feared that people would pre-judge me based on how I looked, talked, or walked, all of which became a reality in my life.

My first experience of mistaken identity played out was when I was six. I recall spending a workday in my dad's transport truck. I was wearing dark clothes, was filthy from top to bottom, and had short hair. At one of our stops I had to use the bathroom. When we entered the office my dad asked the man behind the desk if we could use the restroom. The man said, 'Is it for your son?' My dad replied, 'No, it's for my daughter' (as they both chuckled out loud). The following school year I grew out my hair so I would blend in and avoid situations like that.

Many years later when I was in Grade 8, I recall a friend's younger brother laughing at me as he said that I sounded and looked like a guy. I immediately made every attempt to raise the tone of my voice when speaking for fear that I would be mistaken for a man. It's not that I didn't like men or would have traded my awkward female body for a man's; it was that I didn't like being mistaken for one. These are just two examples of my identity being mistaken. It happens more often than you might think. (It happened again just two days before I wrote this paragraph.) Over time, I have gotten better at laughing it off and not taking it to heart. There is nothing wrong with being a strong, independent woman with short hair and men's clothing.

Whether it's my body image, my weight, my looks, or my choice of clothing and piercings, others will have opinions, that's for sure. I have learned over my lifetime that many people like to categorize things because it makes life easier – on them at any rate. It was years before I could step out from where I was hiding behind that mask and embrace all that I was, no matter what others thought.

I grew up full of confusion, insecurity, and skewed beliefs about myself and my body. I lacked self-love and self-confidence until well into my adult years. I worked hard (and still do) to stay fit, active, and strong, but despite these efforts, I was never satisfied with who I was or what I looked like. It was an inner battle I faced almost daily and one that I longed to move beyond. I just didn't have the tools to move forward, at least not back then.

There was no single, decisive moment in this breakdown, but multiple moments, over the course of many years, before my truth could no longer be suppressed. I reached the point where loving myself and starting the healing process was not only needed, but necessary. Coming to an understanding and place of peace within my body was the first step. The more I understood about myself, the less intense my physical and emotional struggles became. The more I accepted my sexuality and my body, the more my stress diminished and my happiness grew.

The turning point came when I finally decided that my identity was not going to change, and that it didn't need to. What needed to change was my perception of my life and the love I had for myself. I needed to love myself just as I was, so that I could invite others to do the same. It was then that my life began to change for the better.

I came out as a lesbian to my friends and family in 2001. As challenging a time as that was, in the weeks and months to follow the 'back pack" of emotional turmoil I had been carrying around for years grew lighter and lighter. Pent-up emotions around my body image, my sexuality, my desires, shame, guilt, and embarrassment dropped away like 100-pound boulders, each hitting the ground with a thud, signaling the progress of my healing journey.

My self-confidence and self-esteem had been compromised for so long, but no more. I was ready to embrace all aspects of myself, a commitment that still continues to this day.

Self-love is a habit not an attribute.

Something I could not figure out, and still struggle with at times, is that what makes me feel comfortable makes others feel uncomfortable. Why can't we all just live and let live? Love has no bounds and this includes the love we have for ourselves. One of my favourite quotes of all time is by RuPaul (one of the most iconic drag queens you'll ever see): 'If you can't love yourself, how the hell are you going to love somebody else?' This really sums it up.

In order to truly embrace who we are, we must speak our truth, live with authenticity, and practice ways to improve our self-love. Regardless of what others think or say about you or your body, remember that it has everything to do with them, not you. This self-realization was liberating and something I hold close to my heart every day.

Now it's your turn to build your self-confidence through the practices I've taught you. It's your turn to love yourself more than you've ever loved before. Dig deep inside and let go of what's holding you back from being your unique and wonderful self.

Because when you do, it will spill over into all areas of your life and health.

7
_____

THE SYNERGY OF SIX

I believe we are all capable of living a life of vitality and joy. That being said, I understand that life, and a life well-lived, looks different for every person. Each one of us has different experiences, struggles, triumphs, genetics, family backgrounds, personalities, interests, and so on. Regardless of who we are or what our goals are, there will be challenges and times when one of the elements of health feels out of balance. This is all part of learning, growing, and evolving. Just as our bodies strive for homeostasis, so do our minds.

Every single person is going to experience breakdowns along the way to greater health. These breakdowns may relate to your physical, your emotional, your spiritual well-being, or even to all three. My hope is that such breakdowns lead you to some very profound breakthroughs – to turning points that shed light on which course of action is needed next. Breakdowns do not mean you give up. Breakdowns give you feedback and help steer your next steps. They are how you learn and grow, and what propel you forward.

I believe that improvements to overall health are possible at any age and any stage of your life. I'm also convinced that there is a way for everyone to balance these 6 key elements to create the level of well-being you most desire. I know this to be true because I've witnessed it not only in my own life, but in the life of every client I've ever coached.

Living a healthy lifestyle does not need to be difficult, it just needs to be purposeful. It all starts with one small step that propels you from where you are, to where you want to be. What you have learned in this book is no big, cryptic secret. In fact the majority of it is simple common sense. What sets this book apart is its capacity to help you filter out the noise and be guided instead by tried and true strategies.

There are so many companies out there making claims that their product or service works like a magic wand – you're just 'one tap' away from weight loss, vibrancy, and vitality. There is nothing magical about putting my 6 elements of health into play in your life. They cost you nothing. They make no false claims. Yet when you incorporate even one new action step into your life, you will feel the rewards almost immediately. My simple, six-step formula is all it takes to put words into action and gain the momentum and inspiration you need to improve any area of your life: body, mind, and soul.

THE FORMULA

#1 The desire. A desire for change so strong that you will invest the time required to realize it, however long that may be.

#2 The map. It becomes your blueprint and your greatest ally along the journey. On days when you feel you've lost your way, you can look at your map, regroup, and forge onward.

#3 The action. Once you have a map, the next step (and most important one of all) is to take action. The moment you take action is the moment the real transformation happens. Action creates the next ingredient, momentum.

#4 The momentum. Momentum is what keeps you going. You get to build momentum towards what you desire or away from it. The choice is yours.

#5 The consistency. Once the ball is rolling, keep it rolling through consistency. Consistency in your action is what keeps you on track in moments of self-doubt, weakness, or challenge. Consistency is not about perfection or doing something daily without fail. It's more about remembering where you want to go, being kind to yourself, and doing your best.

#6 The belief. By that I mean staying strong and confident in the face of challenges and adversity. Sometimes it might feel like you are taking one step forward and two back. There are going to be days that life takes you off course or your best-laid plans fail. That's life. What's important is that every time you are derailed, you get yourself back on that track. You come back to your core beliefs and return to step #1, your desire, to fuel and propel you.

By making the decision and commitment to make one positive change today will improve your situation. Tomorrow, you will be more motivated to make a second change, and the day after that, a third. Every single step you take in your chosen direction generates momentum for the next step.

This formula can be applied to each and every one of your desires in life and health. Rinse and repeat.

CHOOSE YOUR OWN PATH

Two things will make or break your journey to greater health: your *choices* and your *method*.

You always have a choice. You are the only person responsible for your actions. You cannot place blame on your partner, your kid(s), your family, or something else that in reality is just a way to excuse your behaviour. You are in charge of the choices you make each day. You are the creator of your boundaries. You get to choose what food goes into your body, how much you move each day, the people with whom you surround yourself and every other thing that feeds your mind and spirit. Sure, there are limitations and restrictions that feel beyond your control. For the most part, however, you have the freedom to choose the way you spend your time, what you focus on, and how you live your life.

Next, there's your method. There is always more than one way of doing something. We are all human beings living different experiences. What works for one person may not work for another and that's okay. The important thing is that the decisions you make each day are beneficial to your life. When you make good choices and do things on your terms, in your way, you are more likely to achieve what you desire.

For example, I could tell you that the way to lose your unwanted weight is to go to the gym five days a week for an hour and eat lots of salads for the next six months. But if you hate going to the gym and you don't enjoy eating salad, you are very unlikely to commit to this journey to weight loss. You would not commit because you are not invested in the plan I laid out for you. If instead you forged your own fitness routine and food choices, things you could get behind and commit to, your success would be inevitable.

Too many people live with a 'one-size-fits-all' mentality. They fear that there is only one way to achieve health, and it's got to be difficult and tedious. Some people feel that there are so many insurmountable tasks that they have very little room for personal well-being.

What if you viewed each of the areas you want to change as a stepping stone? When you place one stone and step on it, the momentum gained from that effort will propel you forward to the next. Before you know it, you will have taken many small steps and be well down your path to greater health. To quote Queen Anna of Arendelle, a character in Disney's *Frozen II*, what it comes down to is just 'do the next right thing' – not the next ten right things or next ten steps, just one.

Make a choice today that your future self will thank you for.

The way you integrate each of the elements of health is your choice. When the path you are on is no longer serving you or no longer feels like a 'fit', it's time to choose a new path. Fill your time and your days with routines and rituals that feel good for you, your body, your family situation, and overall lifestyle. And most importantly, choose things you will stick with. If changes feel like a chore, you're not likely to keep doing them.

RIDE THE MOMENTUM

Physics recognizes two factors that affect momentum: mass and velocity. If we look at momentum as it relates to the 6 elements of health, mass refers to the importance or weight you give the self-improvement in question, and velocity is the direction of that choice.

If the change you imagine is of little importance to you and your overall lifestyle, you are not likely to gain much momentum in that direction. By contrast, if you are fully committed and downright determined to make a change, you will. It's pretty simple. If taking a certain action means achieving a better quality of life – less aches and pains, more energy, vitality, and a longer life in which to play and enjoy your kids or grandkids – I would hazard to guess you are more likely to create positive momentum.

As you gain momentum you begin to pick up speed. The faster you travel in the direction that you want to go, the greater your velocity. Velocity can either drive you deeper into a downward spiral, or it can propel you upward in the direction of your desires. Once you start to gain velocity in the direction of greater health, the faster you will take each step on the way to that destination. Where attention goes, energy will flow.

All it takes is a single step in the right direction to gain momentum.

Creating momentum as it relates to the elements of health might look like this. Say you make the decision to walk for five minutes today and add on one minute each day for the next 21 days. In less than a month, you will be able to walk for over 30 minutes straight. Having gained positive momentum from one small action, then adding a little more effort each day to follow, before you know it, you end up with what amounts to great strides.

Apply the same strategy to any aspect of your health that you want to improve. Want to make a practice of meditation? Start with two minutes of deep breathing, then add one minute each day until you reach your intended goal. Want to eat more veggies? Start by adding a half cup more vegetables to your plate each day until you get to your goal. Want to reduce the time you spend on your phone? Commit to one hour of screen-free time each evening, then extend that time by 15 minutes each week thereafter. You get the idea.

By taking the end goal and breaking it down into manageable, bite-sized pieces, you generate momentum in the right direction. From simple, seemingly innocuous changes, you create stepping stones that steadily propel you closer to your goal.

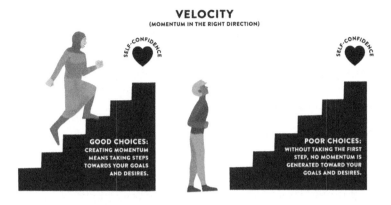

HABITUAL LAYERING

We all have habits that we can do practically with our eyes closed. You know the ones I mean: brushing your teeth, combing your hair, going to and from work, making coffee, or the place you put your keys upon arriving home. These are things we do so often, they become a part of our day that requires little or no thought. Some of these habits increase our health, some detract from it, and some have no effect either way.

No wonder changing old habits or creating new ones is so hard. You are having to create and ingrain a new brain pattern. That is why it always pays to have a map that shows how you are going to get from A to B. A map helps to take out the guesswork and keep you on track while still providing room for new opportunities and deviation if needed.

In order to make lasting, sustainable change without becoming overwhelmed and paralyzed, it's important to focus on one thing at a time. Not five things, just one. When you put too much pressure on yourself, or try to make too many changes all at once, you are more likely to end up feeling frustrated, defeated, and unable to follow through on any of the changes. This leads to the 'been-there-done-that-never-worked' mindset. It becomes a self-fulfilling prophecy.

By taking time to map out and set small, achievable intentions over the course of days, weeks, or months, you hold yourself accountable, reduce the likelihood of being overwhelmed by circumstances or expectations, and increase your likelihood of success. By taking a big goal and breaking it down into bite-sized pieces, you make the goal feel more achievable.

Let's say, you want to start exercising three days a week to prepare your body for a five-kilometre run six months from now. Without 1) a clear schedule of your workouts, 2) a plan for the focus of each training session, 3) how long those sessions will be, 4) what you should eat and when, and 5) a realistic timeline to get you from where you are to your bigger goal, you are far less likely to succeed.

But with a clear vision, even on days when you are feeling uninspired, tired, or down-right lazy, you can whip open your planner, remind yourself what you're working for, drag your butt out the door, and make it happen. Writing down your goals and objectives is a great tool. You can do this using a day-timer, an online calendar, journal, or notebook. Keeping a record of your accomplishments will also give you something to look back on, so you know what went well, and what you would do differently next time.

Your ability to commit to one small thing that improves your health means you have the ability to commit to 100.

I hope this book leaves you feeling inspired, like anything is possible, and eager to take action in your life. I want you to feel in charge, confident, and motivated. But please, do not try to overhaul every aspect of your health at the same time.

Stacking a bunch of changes on your plate all at once is a recipe for feeling unstable, that your life is changing 'too much, too fast'.

Give each change time to take root before adding more, so healthy habits can 'grow on you'.

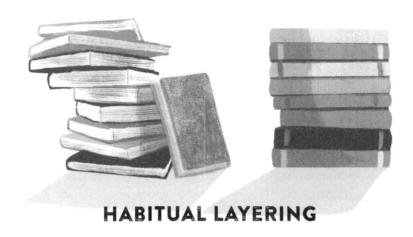

HABITUAL LAYERING

When you 'layer' habits, you put one on top of the other in an organized fashion. Otherwise, you jumble them together, and that's when things can become messy and overwhelming.

Some habits might be easy to change and only take days to become routine. Others are going to take months. Making improvements to any area of your life takes time and patience. But when you layer on one new habit or one new way of living at a time, it has a chance to become part of your day and your routines. It has the ability to become part of your life, ingrained, and 'your norm'. Once that happens, then and only then do you add the next layer of change, confident that it too shall succeed.

By implementing one small change and committing to it until it becomes habitual, you make the process of change easier, attainable, and sustainable. This is what I like to call *habitual layering**. What matters is not how long it takes, but your level of consistency and commitment to the process.

. . .

TAP INTO YOUR MOTIVATION

Motivation is something I have always had in plenty. Unfortunately, I can't even give it away, much less mass-produce it. What I can offer are the strategies I use to tap into my motivation, to help you tap into yours.

But first, I want to talk a little about what motivation actually is. According to Kendra Cherry, a psychosocial rehabilitation specialist, motivation is activated by several factors. Biological, emotional, social, and cognitive behaviours activate our level of motivation. These motivations can be either intrinsic or extrinsic.

Intrinsic motivation is when you do something because it's personally rewarding to you. For example, if you are passionate about playing softball, you easily show up each week ready to go with a fun and positive vibration. Extrinsic motivation, on the other hand, is when you do something to earn a reward, recognition, or to avoid punishment. These are times when you do something that personally you would rather not, but are willing to carry out in exchange for this external benefit.

Motivation explains why a person acts or does the things they do. It is the driving force behind our actions. What leads us to get a drink of water? We're thirsty. What motivates us to call a friend? We're lonely and in need of connection. What leads us to meditate? We want to feel grounded and calm.

Many theorists of motivation maintain that it is something that is learned and fostered in childhood. It comes back to the concept of encouraging versus forcing. There's a fine line between encouraging people (both kids and adults) to do something, and forcing them. Can you recall moments in your childhood when you were forced to do things that you did not want to do? Your level of motivation was low or sometimes non-existent. Yet, the times you were inspired and gently encouraged to make something happen, you did so and it felt good. Your self-motivation kicked in and you accomplished something with pride and satisfaction.

If you have ever had the desire to run a marathon or lose 25 pounds, you know full well that desire alone will not enable you to make it a reality. Turning desire into a goal and then actually following through on that goal requires motivation. Your motivation is what keeps you going despite all the obstacles, challenges, and setbacks you meet along the way.

Become crystal clear about what you desire and why you want it, and the motivation will follow.

From a psychological perspective, there are three main ingredients in motivation: activation, persistence, and intensity. I believe there is a fourth key ingredient, our *feelings*. In order to tap into our motivation, the first thing we need to do is decide how we want to feel. Our feelings drive our behaviours. When we can describe how we want to feel, we can reverse engineer and make a plan to attract those feelings.

After we know how we want to feel (our ultimate physical desire), the next step is *activation*. Activation involves initiating a behaviour. This could be hiring a coach, signing up for an exercise program, or buying a gym membership. This is when you take action to achieve what you want. Once you activate your desire you can move onto the next step, persistence.

Persistence is the ongoing energy you put into your desire, regardless of the obstacles that you face. For example, hiring a health coach may come with some perceived obstacles. You don't know what to expect because you've never had a coach or mentor before. It's a big investment and you're not sure how you will pay for it. It brings up feelings of uncertainty or failure because you think you 'should' be able to do things on your own. You fear it will be too time-consuming and you're already feeling maxed out. The barriers between you and what you desire are real, but persistence means you keep going no matter what, even if you make only the smallest progress for days on end. If you want something bad enough you will find the money, make the time, and tap into your inner drive to make it happen.

The final ingredient is *intensity*. This refers to the concentration and energy you invest in realizing your desire. You might be the kind of person who joins a group program with good intentions but within weeks you find yourself doing the bare minimum. Someone who has more intensity gets as much out of the coaching as possible, stays focused, asks questions, and is willing to share wins and challenges. Intensity does not mean going full throttle every single day. It just means you are engaged and want to get the most out of the situation.

Here are some tips to tap into your motivation:

- Ask yourself two questions: "How do I want to feel in my body?" and "What can I do that will get me there?"
- Set goals around things that really matter to you. They will be the source of your motivation.
- Reflect on your life and a time when you achieved something you really wanted. Use that to fuel your future endeavours.
- If the goal is big, break it into bite-sized pieces. Small things done repeatedly add up to big things over time.
- Make a plan that includes a schedule. It will show you how you intend to get from where you are right now (Point A) to where you want to go (Point B). It should be realistic but challenging, while still requiring you to be consistent, so you can hold yourself accountable. For example, a plan could be a daily walk over a distance that increases from week to week so you slowly improve your speed or endurance. If the goal is too hard at the onset you are not likely to commit to it. If it's too easy you are not going to make the progress you're looking for.

- Remind yourself that it took time (months, years, decades) to get where you are right now, and it's going to take time to get where you want to go. Be patient and kind.
- Avoid comparing yourself to others. Your journey and process are your own and the way you get to your desire is motivated by an inner knowing, not an external factor.
- Don't lose sight of your answers to those first two questions. They are the reasons you are doing this in the first place. They make it matter.
- Visualize where you want to be, what you want to look like, who you want to hang with, how you want to eat, etc. Take yourself there. There is power in visualization!
- Reward your efforts with something other than food! Celebrate the small wins because they lead to big victories.

Think about how you want to feel in your body (*movement*), in your mind (*mindfulness*), your level of energy (*nutrition*), your sense of belonging (*connection*), your mental clarity and physical body (*rest*), and your confidence (*self-love*). Attach a feeling to your desires and dreams because that is the first step to finding your motivation.

Since motivation is driven by feelings, take action to generate the feelings that will help keep you motivated. When I want to feel grounded and calm, I meditate. When I want to feel creative and inspired, I walk. When I want to feel connected and loved, I call my mom or my siblings. When I want to feel strong and energized, I exercise. And, when I want to feel healthy and happy, I eat fresh veggies.

Motivation, learned or not, has the power to change you. If you work backwards from the feeling you want to accomplish, you can see what action is needed to get you there. Your core beliefs about yourself inform the thoughts you have, those thoughts motivate your actions, and those actions create results.

In therapy this is viewed as the triangle effect. One side of the triangle is directly related to the other two sides. Your *thoughts* decide your *actions*, and your actions propel your *feelings*. Once this cycle is established, you continue to see results which continue to propel you in a positive direction along your journey.

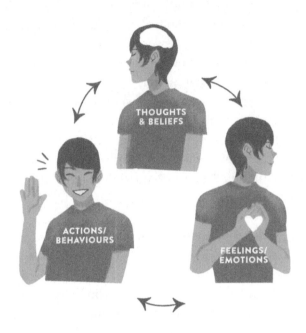

For instance, perhaps your desire is to gain strength. You know that gaining strength won't happen on hope and prayer alone. A feeling has to be attached to the desire, and an action needs to be taken to get you closer to that desire. Physical strength is built on consistency and positive thinking. This in turn drives those good feelings, so you continue to take action toward what you most desire.

EMBRACING CHANGE

There are a few things in life that are guaranteed, and change is one of them. It happens all the time, in many facets of your life and many times when you least expect it or want it. It's also easy to get set in your ways and complacent. For many people, just the thought of change makes the heart race, palms sweat, and internal radar go off. But worrying about change, whether you are experiencing it or anticipating it, is a waste of precious resources. It's far better to reframe how you feel about and how you approach change. When you approach change as if it's happening 'for you', not 'to you', you are able to free up your energy to best deal with the task at hand.

Reframing is also important when you initiate changes to your lifestyle. It is only possible to make lasting change after you admit that your current circumstances are no longer serving you. Having done that, you become more self-aware and your ability to change your circumstances becomes stronger. You come to know with all your being that you are ready, willing, and able to make lasting change happen.

This analogy reminds me a lot of Alcoholics Anonymous (AA). Nobody can make someone go to AA, clean up their lifestyle, and commit to a healthier and more self-loving path. They must want it, believe it's possible, and worth it, and they must take action all on their own. That's exactly how it went for my client Liz.

Liz had been very inactive for about 20 years. She had taken to reading, watching TV, and puttering about in her pool. Her desire to be active was very low. She walked once in a while but never stretched or did any type of weight-bearing activity. She liked the way her life was and didn't see a reason to change it despite her husband's ongoing nudges.

Her husband, a client of mine for over two years, wanted nothing more than his wife to be more active and strong. He feared for her loss of bone density and her risk of falling. But the change had to come from Liz. No amount of comments or encouragement from her husband would work.

One day, Liz decided it was time, all on her own. She made the decision to change her lifestyle on her terms and timeline. I believe that is the only reason she has stuck with her weekly routine and is continuing to see progress.

IT'S NEVER ALL OR NOTHING

If there's one popular notion that rubs me the wrong way, it's that something must be done fully and completely or it's 'pointless'. In fact, rather than prompt people to decisive, committed action, that outlook is more likely to discourage them from ever doing anything at all.

In life there are areas of grey. If you're anything like me, you do not enjoy the grey. Regardless, it exists. There is a middle ground for most things and we have to remember that doing something is always better than doing nothing. 'All or nothing' simply does not apply where health is concerned.

At first, implementing new routines and new ways of moving through the day might require compromise, communication with your family, and adjustments to your current schedule. It might mean juggling a few things or getting creative with your thinking. Making a hard and fast commitment to do something, like to stop eating chips (even though you *love* chips), sets you up for failure. When you inevitably sit down to enjoy some chips it's likely to go very poorly. The craving will be strong, overindulgence will creep in, and you are likely to leave the scene feeling defeated and as if you failed.

Let's reframe that thinking pattern right now. There is no 'all or nothing'. Eating chips a few times a month is part of a healthy diet. Yes, it's true. Eating things you enjoy is part of living. Life events will unfold, such as parties, gatherings, and movie nights, at which you can enjoy those chips without guilt or feelings of defeat or deprivation.

The same is true about starting a new morning routine that involves ten minutes of meditation and ten minutes of stretching. Just because you miss a morning here or there because you woke up to a sick kid or you slept in and had less time doesn't mean you're off track or that you've failed. Committing to something and seeing it through does not outlaw flexibility or compromise. You can always reset, restart, and reframe.

Only one person has the power to change your beliefs, and that person is you.

You do not need to take resolute action in terms of all 6 elements to live a happier and healthier life. That's not what this book is about. It's to enable you to decide which areas need more attention, where you want to start, to be kind with yourself and your process, and take action wherever possible. Reframe any 'all or nothing' thinking you may have into something more positive, that allows you to deviate at times from the plan, without dropping it completely.

BALANCE THE HEXAGON

If you're like most people, there are a few elements that you naturally gravitate towards. They become a regular part of your life without much effort. To demonstrate, I will use the inverted triangle example I shared with you in the Introduction. I have no problem getting daily exercise, eating three cups of vegetables each day, ensuring I get enough rest, and staying connected with my family and friends. I do them without thinking. The elements that require more of my attention are mindfulness and self-love. Going back to your inverted triangle, you know which areas of your health are habitual and which need more attention. You know which elements are the strongest parts of your hexagon.

I'm sure you would agree, it's not that you don't care about *all* areas of your health, it's more likely that you must devote more attention to certain areas in order to make them a priority ... and then, of course, to take action. It's about striking a balance between each element to keep the integrity of the whole. A lopsided hexagon has less stability, and less ability to withstand any stress and pressure that is placed on it.

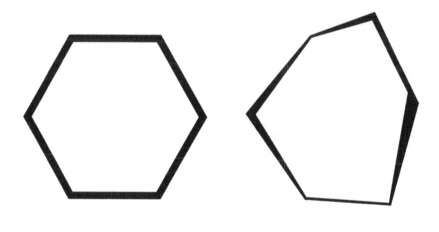

Keeping balance in your life means giving equal focus to each part of the whole.

That is exactly how I view health and well-being. If one area of life is extremely out of balance for too long, we get sick or injured. We suffer from things like depression, extreme mood swings, chronic pain, loneliness, resentment, and so on. I believe that the more we are able to balance each element of our health, the better balanced we will be as individuals.

Now that you know which of the 6 elements are your *bright spots**
and which could use a bit more attention, you can move forward
to creating balance. Some things will be more challenging to
implement and require a bit more effort and focus. Start small,
breathe deeply, stay consistent, be kind to yourself, and over time
your hexagon's structure will become balanced and integrated.

Achieving balance in your hexagon might take months or even
years. It's a journey and a process. It takes time and requires little
adjustments along the way. The best part is that one day you will
look back and realize how far you've come. That will be the
moment you awaken to the possibilities that still lie ahead. If you
can change one thing, you can change ten.

I cannot stress more the importance of celebrating what you're
doing well and then deciding on your next step. By celebrating
your wins and your bright spots along the way, you lean into those
good feelings that help you gain confidence and momentum for
the next area of growth. This is how the hexagon achieves
balance, and so do you.

SYNERGIZE YOUR HEALTH

I've shared the science and the strategies. I've also shared stories
from clients and my own health journey. I have opened up about
my home life as a child, my brother's medical concerns, my view
of Western Medicine, and my transition to more natural living.
I've shared my struggles with body image, my eating disorder, and
my intrigue with food and nutrition.

I believe that our career path and interests are greatly influenced
by our own life experiences. We are drawn into a certain field of
study, be it a hobby or our life's work, because that's what we need
for healing. And then, once we learn how to support and improve
our own lives we want to help others do the same. That's my story.
I want to make a difference in the lives of the people I touch,

through what I know, what I've learned, and what I've come to understand about well-being. The health challenges we face as individuals have the ability to change us if we're ready, willing, and able. Are you ready, willing, and able to develop new routines and make small changes that will improve the quality of your life?

Like me, I know you have your unique story and life path that have been sprinkled with triumphs and tribulations. Those are the things that make us human. My story is no worse or better than yours, it's just different. I encourage you, as you move forward on your health journey, to look at setbacks (previous and future) as gifts. They are there to teach, remind, and invoke change if you are willing to see them in that light.

Each and every experience in life teaches you something. I urge you to take your health and well-being into your own hands and start implementing changes right now. View the changes you desire as gifts that you're giving to yourself. Taking your health into your own hands is the best gift you can give. No matter what kind of habit you choose to tackle first, decide on it, commit to it, and do it.

It will take time and effort. Some days will be easier and others more challenging but take things one day at a time. It's fine to have the long view of where you want to go in mind, but remember the short view is more manageable. The short view and the daily choices add up and lead you to that long vision.

I can give you all the tools and strategies you need to develop a healthier lifestyle, but the thing I cannot give you is the motivation. That has to come from within. That has to come from a place inside of you that wants the change more than you want to live in your current circumstances. Making change today that your future self will appreciate has to be more powerful than staying stuck and settling for feeling 'okay'.

I believe that in order to live our greatest life we need to synergize our health. That means giving attention to each of six elements: rest, movement, connection, nutrition, mindfulness, and self-love.

When we do, the sum of these elements produces a greater sense of vitality and joy than each can on its own.

Embarking on a new way of creating greater health and making changes is not always easy, but it is worth it. I know, I've made many over my lifetime and continue to. If you truly want to live my 6 elements of health you cannot just read about them, listen to me speak, or watch me on video. You have to live them. The moment you take action is the moment you will create the habits and feel a difference, in mind, body, and spirit.

I will leave you with this final thought,

Well-being cannot be measured by a number, nor is it a place you arrive at. It's a way of life.

WORKS CITED

American Addiction Centers. (n.d.). *Women's Body Image and BMI: 100 Years in the US*. Retrieved October 12, 2020, from https://www.rehabs.com/explore/womens-body-image-and-bmi/

Ball, P. (2016, April 07). Why Nature Prefers Hexagons - Issue 35: Boundaries. Retrieved January 30, 2021, from https://nautil.us/issue/35/boundaries/why-nature-prefers-hexagons

Berardi, J. (2017). *The Essentials of Sport and Exercise Nutrition: Certification Manual*. Precision Nutrition, Inc.

Betuel, E. (2019, April 23). *How Much Time Does the Average Person Spend Sitting? Reports Show It's Dramatically Changing*. Inverse. http://www.inverse.com/article/55165-time-spent-sitting-average-person

Bunn, M. (2019, November 1). Forest Bathing, Earthing and Nature Immersion. *Thrive Global*. Retrieved November 15, 2020, from http://thriveglobal.com/stories/forest-bathing-earthing-and-nature-immersion/

Centers for Disease Control & Prevention. (2016, February 16). *1 In 3 Adults Don't Get Enough Sleep*. Retrieved October 12, 2020, from http://www.cdc.gov/media/releases/2016/p0215-enough-sleep.html

Cherry, K. (2020, January 15). *Differences of Extrinsic and Intrinsic Motivation*. verywellmind. Retrieved November 23, 2020, from https://www.verywellmind.com/differences-between-extrinsic-and-intrinsic-motivation-2795384

Go Paleo. (2019, November). *Unplugging + Connecting*. 60-63.

How Technology Impacts Sleep Quality. (2020, October 21). Retrieved January 17, 2021, from https://www.sleep.org/ways-technology-affects-sleep/

Howard, J. (2018, March 9). The Ever-Changing 'Ideal' of Female Beauty. *CNN Health*. Retrieved October 11, 2020, from https://www.cnn.com/2018/03/07/health/body-image-history-of-beauty-explainer-intl/index.html

Hudnall, M. (2018, June 10). Try Body Neutrality When Body Positivity Seems Impossible. *Fitwoman*. http://www.fitwoman.-com/blog/body-neutrality-2/

Huffington, A. S. (2017). *The Sleep Revolution: Transforming Your Life, One Night at a Time*. Harmony Books.

Kozicka, P. (2015, May 29). 1 in 5 Canadian Women Not Satisfied With Their Appearance: Survey. *Global News*. http://globalnews.ca/news/2025789/1-in-5-canadian-women-not-satisfied-with-their-appearance-survey

Li, Q. (2018, May 01). The Benefits of 'Forest Bathing'. Retrieved January 25, 2021, from https://time.com/5259602/japanese-forest-bathing/

Lopez, A. (2016, July 18). Mindset vs. Mindfulness. Retrieved January 28, 2021, from https://www.mindheart-space.-com/post/2016/07/17/mindset-vs-mindfulness

Mead, E. (2020, September 1). *The History and Origin of Meditation*. PositivePsychology.com. http://positivepsychology.com/history-of-meditation/

Merriam-Webster. (n.d.) Body Image. In *Merriam-Webster.com Medical Dictionary.com*. Retrieved November 27, 2020, from http://www.merriam-webster.com/medical/body%20image

Morgan, C. (2015, March 9). 16 Truths About Real Love. *Huff-Post*. http://www.huffpost.com/entry/16-characteristics-of-real-love_b_6237802?guccounter=1

National Eating Disorders Association. (2018, February 22). *Body Image*. http://www.nationaleatingdisorders.org/body-image-0

National Geographic. (2017, April 10). *5 "Blue Zones" Where the World's Healthiest People Live*. http://www.nationalgeographic.com/books/features/5-blue-zones-where-the-worlds-healthiest-people-live/

Newsonen, S. (2015, February 26). Love Yourself Before You Love Others. *Psychology Today*. http://www.psychologytoday.com/us/blog/the-path-passionate-happiness/201502/love-your-self-you-love-others

Nature's Fare Markets. (2020, September/October). Body Neutrality, A Gentle Approach To How We Think About Our Bodies. *The Good Life*. 21-22. Retrieved November 15, 2020 from https://issuu.com/naturesfaremarkets/docs/nfm_the-goodlife_septoct2020_lores/s/10912755

Olson, E. J. (2019, June 6). How Many Hours of Sleep Do You Need? *Mayo Clinic*. http://www.mayoclinic.org/healthy-life-style/adult-health/expert-answers/how-many-hours-of-sleep-are-enough/faq-20057898

Oxford Dictionary. (n.d.). Body image. In *Oxford Learners' Dictionaries*. Retrieved November 15, 2020, from https://www.oxfordlearnersdictionaries.com/us/definition/english/body-image?q=body+image

ParticipAction. (2018). *ParticipAction Pulse Report*. 4. https://participaction.cdn.prismic.io/participaction%2F55d68455-6812-437a-

853a-54c5458a314e_participaction-pulse-report-powered-by-mec-en.pdf

Petty, A. (2020, February 12). *How Men's Perfect Body Types Have Changed Throughout History*. The List. Retrieved October 11, 2020, from https://www.thelist.com/56105/mens-perfect-body-types-changed-throughout-history/

Petty, A. (2018, May 2). *How Women's 'Perfect' Body Types Changed Throughout History.* The List. Retrieved October 11, 2020, from https://www.thelist.com/44261/womens-perfect-body-types-changed-throughout-history/

Ranadive, A. (2016, March 24). *Fixed v. Growth Mindset.* Medium. http://medium.com/leadership-motivation-and-impact/fixed-v-growth-mindset-902e7d0081b3

Robbins, M. (2019). *Summary: The 5 second rule.* Monee, IL: EpicRead.

Segar, M. (2015). *No Sweat: How the Simple Science of Motivation Can Bring You a Lifetime of Fitness.* AMACOM.

Statistics Canada. (2015, November 27). *Adult Obesity Prevalence in Canada and the United States.* http://www150.statcan.gc.-ca/n1/pub/82-625-x/2011001/article/11411-eng.htm

Fisher-Titus Healthy Living Team. (2018, September 18). *The Effects of Technology on Mental Health.* Fisher Titus. http://www.fishertitus.org/health/effects-technology-mental-health

World Health Organization. (2018, February 23). *Physical Activity.* Retrieved October 12, 2020, from http//www.who.int/newsroom/fact-sheets/detail/physical-activity

World Health Organization. (2019, October 17). *Childhood Overweight and Obesity.* Retrieved October 3, 2020, from https://www.who.int/dietphysicalactivity/childhood/en/

World Health Organization. (2020, March 27). *Mental health and Psychological Resilience During the COVID-19 Pandemic.* Retrieved

October 3, 2020, from https://www.euro.who.int/en/health-topics/health-emergencies/coronavirus-covid-19/news/news/2020/3/mental-health-and-psychological-resilience-during-the-covid-19-pandemic

KRISTY'S HEALTH DEFINITIONS

Body Image: Body image is the way we see ourselves based on our physical appearance. It can be based on how we look, our body shape, size and how we compare ourselves to others. It's what we see when we look in the mirror and those things can be positive or negative. It's how we carry ourselves each day, how we dress, our hair style, choice of make-up, piercings, and tattoos. Body image is our self-expression.

Body neutrality: Body neutrality means focusing on all the great things you can do instead of being consumed by your looks. It's a process that helps to shift your thinking around your body from the negative to the positive. It frees up energy you might be wasting putting yourself down or blocking yourself from doing or trying something you want to do because of how you look. By embracing this philosophy you shift your focus from what's impossible for you to what's possible, with less judgement and shame.

Bookending: "Bookending your day" is an expression I use to represent the rituals or routines you use each day to set you up for success. Spending time each morning and each evening doing something mindful and intentional sets you up for success in life, love and career and it is also a great way to promote self-aware-ness and confidence.

Bright Spots: Bright spots are those moments, experiences, and silver linings that shine through during even the darkest, most challenging times. They remind you that there is good in the world, and there is something to learn and appreciate in any situa-tion. Look for the bright spots because they exist if you're open to seeing them.

Diet: Diet simply means eating foods that are necessary for our survival. Diet is not about deprivation, elimination or restriction but about nourishment, choosing whole foods and eating mother nature's bounty. Dieting is not a way of life but eating a whole foods, low processed diet is.

Downtime: Downtime is that time when we are lost in daydream, creative projects and our imagination is flowing. It's a time when we are fully immersed in a single task without stress or urgency. It's the space between.

Earthing: Earthing is planting your feet, spreading your toes, and feeling the gentle embrace of mother earth below. It provides you with a sense of calm, sacredness, and security. It's one of the best ways to ground your mind and spirit when you feel you've drifted off course. Earthing gives your body energy and vitality like nothing else ever can.

Emotional Eating: Emotional eating is choosing food in moments of fear, loneliness, stress, overwhelm or sadness to achieve a more comforting feeling. It's a way to fill a void that you feel in your body or your mind. In most cases, it's something learned from childhood or early adulthood. I believe that eating in and of itself is emotional. Food carries a charge, a memory, feel-ings, emotions or triggers. Eating can be a way of avoiding some other area of your life that needs a little more attention. Emotions are a part of being human, embrace them and feel them.

Excuses: Excuses are things you say or do to avoid discomfort, pain, confrontation or failure. They are like boulders you drop in your own way that stop you from taking the next step on life's journey. Excuses are a way to justify your choices but they hold you back from progressing, trying, learning and growing. Let go of your excuses and watch the shifts that happen in your life.

Forest Bathing: Forest bathing means walking among the trees, breathing in their scent, inhaling their fresh clean air, and honouring their beauty. Bathing among the trees is a way to wash off and let go of what is no longer serving you and causing you stress. It's a physical, mental and emotional reset. It grounds you.

Food Products: Food products are those foods that come in a box or package and have been highly processed, contain preservatives, and ingredients you don't know or cannot pronounce. Food products generally have long lists of ingredients and are void of nutrients for growth and overall health. They may give the illusion that they are 'healthy' simple choices but most food products do not come from the earth or the farm and therefore are less than optimal options.

Habitual Layering: Habitual layering is taking one small action, doing it consistently over time, making it a habit and then layering on the next habit, using the same blueprint. Layering one good habit onto another creates momentum, it puts action behind thought and it creates time and space for life long lasting change. Habitual layering creates progress and progress creates results.

Element: With regards to health, an element represents the framework by which a life of vitality and joy are created. Each element represents an integral part of the whole. When the elements of REST, CONNECTION, MOVEMENT, NUTRI-

TION, MINDFULNESS & SELF-LOVE, are given equal attention, they create a tapestry; this is well-being.

Recovery: Recovery is about down time, rest and sound sleep. It's giving your body time to repair, rejuvenate and recover. It is when your body goes to work to clean up the damage from the world around you, from exercise and most importantly, when your immune system goes to work to keep you healthy.

Rules: Rules are put in place to protect us, to help gain control, and to keep order. Some rules we invoke ourselves as a way of protecting us and those we love from harm or failure. Growing up, rules are in place to help us make sense of the word, to provide consistency and predictability (which provides us with physical and emotional safety). As an adult, some rules are put in place by others and when they do not align with our values and beliefs we have to forge our own path and create our own course. Some rules are just meant to be broken.

Self-Care: Self-care is carving out time each day for the things that bring you joy, make you feel your best and put a smile on your face. Self-care is about a feeling. Doing the things that evoke feelings of excitement, inspiration, passion, relaxation or calmness in your body. It's an internal knowing that what you are doing is needed for your health and happiness.

Self-Awareness: Self-awareness is connection with source energy. It's an understanding of what is needed in your life and the life of those around you. It's a state of mind and a tuning into how your actions impact your life, your families, your friends and the world at large.

Success: Success can take many forms. It cannot be measured but felt from within. Success is about feeling accomplished, inspired, motivated and like you have arrived. It's about taking action on the journey that takes you from here to there. It's what you learn on that journey and what you do with what you have learned.

Synergize: Synergy is when one or more elements interact to produce a joint effect greater than the effects they could achieve separately. To *synergize your health* means you give attention to each element (rest, movement, connection, nutrition, mindfulness & self-love) and when you do, the sum of these elements produces a greater sense of vitality and joy than they can on their own.

ACKNOWLEDGMENTS

This book would not have been possible without all the special people in my world. I'm grateful to those who have touched my life, broken me down, and built me up. To those who have been there with me through the challenges and the triumphs. To all those who have crossed my path, impacted my growth, taught me valuable life lessons, and continue to.

FLORA: My wife who's been there through the tears, the laughter, the challenges, and the triumphs. This book would not have been possible without your gentle but firm encouragement to find joy in reading. Reading led me to writing! I would not be doing the things I'm doing today without your ongoing inspiration, guidance, unconditional love, and endless support. Together we're an unstoppable force and I know we're destined to leave this world a better place.

GRIFFYN: For your daily reminders to have fun, laugh, and find happiness in all life's little moments. For your energy, sense of humour, smile, hugs, kisses, and the love you bring to my life everyday. I am truly blessed to call you my son.

MOM & DAD: Together we have shared many wonderful and challenging times. The best part is that no matter what, we've always found our way back to the true meaning of family, and for that I am forever grateful. You have stood by me even when my choices and decisions did not make sense to you. You continue to shower my family and I with love and eternal connection, despite the physical distance between us.

ASHLEY: My sister, for listening, caring, supporting, and sharing an unbreakable bond that is never taken for granted. To you and **CRAIG** for making me an auntie to two wonderful nieces. You are not just my sister but a forever friend.

RICHARD: My brother, my strength. For teaching me compassion, unconditional love, tenacity, resilience, and the importance of family. You're an inspiration in my life and always will be.

ANNE & GERRY: My wonderful in-laws. For caring for Griffyn so I could write. For all your support, heartfelt conversations, and outdoor adventures.

AUNT JO: For your ongoing acceptance, wholehearted conversations, and love. Your door has always remained open and so has your heart. You've been like a second mother to me and you will always have a special place in my heart.

AUNT JANINE: For reading my manuscript and helping me weave it into something beautiful. You're an inspiration, someone I admire, look up to, and appreciate with all my heart.

DON: For all your edits. You took my ideas, my concepts, and my words, and brought them to life.

NIKKI: For all your amazing design work and tech support.

KIM V: For your teachings and your friendship. For taking the time to read my manuscript and write my forward. I'm honoured.

MICHELLE S: For taking the time to connect with me, read my manuscript, and review my book. You're an inspiration in my life and my work.

ANITA: First and foremost, for helping me rid myself of all the years of unnecessary baggage I was carrying. It was weighing me down and holding me back. Thank you for helping me learn to trust myself, spread my wings, and move forth with courage. And, as of late, for becoming a friend. Our time together has been a pivotal part of my life's journey.

GRAMA FLO: For always believing in me, allowing me to be myself when others didn't, and for showering me with love, two armed hugs I never wanted to end, and for all the foot rubs a girl could ask for.

AUNT BETTY: For ensuring I never went without. You provided care, food, a place to land, hope, support, and love to my family at the times when we needed it the most.

DIANE, JENNIFER, CHRISTINE, ROSA, DR. ENTNER, KATHY, MURPHY & DOMINICK: For reading my manuscript and providing me with such heartfelt reviews and valuable feedback. I'm eternally grateful.

JENNIFER SPARKS: For your layout and formatting expertise. And most of all, for making my book look so freaking fantastic!

MY CLIENTS: For letting me be a part of your health journey and sharing your success stories in this book.

I am thankful for my community and my friends far and wide.

I am thankful for my softball team, the ISOTOPES. You know who you are.

I am thankful for each and every life experience that has brought me to where I am today.

And thank **YOU**, the person who is holding this book, learning from my strategies, and implementing my tools.

With deepest gratitude,

Kristy

RESOURCES

All resources can be found by going to: kristyware.com/6-elements-resources/

The 6 Elements of Health Workbook
Download your guide to creating greater vitality and joy!
This workbook is jam packed with simple strategies to help you implement each of the elements into your life, additional information for each element, and 'habit hexagons' to help keep you on track.

REST
Rest & Recovery Guide
Your free guide to rest, recovery, better sleep, and more energy!

MOVEMENT
Restore Your Core Guide (for women)
Free guide that shares 5 Tips to help you regain core strength at any stage of life.

Reclaiming Your Core Confidence Self-Study Program (for all genders)
The 8 week program designed to increase your core strength and reduce back and hip pain so you can get back to doing what you love, without doing sit-ups or crunches, ever!
Includes 4 progressive mini workouts and a stretch routine.

CONNECTION
Quiz
What's your self-care synergy level?
Take this 5 minute free quiz to discover more about yourself, what elements of your health you've got dialed, and which ones could use a little more attention. Be sure to share this with your friends and family! When we are more connected to ourselves we become more connected to those around us and mother nature.

NUTRITION
Snacking Survival Guide
This free guide provides you with body positive solutions to the common struggle of evening snacking.

Meal Planning eBooks (gluten-free & vegetarian options)

MINDFULNESS
Synergize Your Day Affirmations Card Deck

Each of the quotes you read sprinkled throughout this book have been put into a daily affirmations card deck.

SELF-LOVE
Vibrantly Confident Self-study Program (for women) ~
The 3-part video program to help you develop more self-acceptance, make peace with your body, and turn your triggers into your triumphs.

PLEASE LEAVE A REVIEW

The best thing you can do to help independent authors like myself is to give an honest and heartfelt review.

If you enjoyed this book, please go to Amazon.com or Amazon.ca and leave a review. It would mean so much, and help me reach more readers. Thank you!